Recent Results in Cancer Research 98

Perioperative Chemotherapy

Rationale, Risk and Results

Edited by

U. Metzger F. Largiadèr H.-J. Senn

With 48 Figures and 45 Tables

Springer-Verlag
Berlin Heidelberg New York Tokyo

Proceedings of an International Symposium,
17/18 March 1983, Zurich University Hospital

Dr. Urs Metzger
Chirurgische Onkologie
Departement Chirurgie
Universitätsklinik
8091 Zürich, Switzerland

Professor Dr. Felix Largiadèr
Departement Chirurgie
Universitätsklinik
8091 Zürich, Switzerland

Professor Dr. Hans-Jörg Senn
Kantonsspital St. Gallen
Medizinische Klinik C
9007 St. Gallen, Switzerland

Sponsored by the Swiss League against cancer

ISBN-13: 978-3-642-82434-0 e-ISBN-13: 978-3-642-82432-6
DOI: 10.1007/978-3-642-82432-6

Library of Congress Cataloging in Publication Data. Main entry under title: Perioperative chemotherapy. (Recent results in cancer research; 98). Proceedings of the "Perioperative Chemotherapy" Symposium, held 17/18 March 1983 at the Zurich University Hospital. Includes bibliographies and index. 1. Cancer-Adjuvant treatment-Congresses. 2. Metastasis-Prevention-Congresses. I. Metzger, U. (Urs), 1945- . II. Largiadèr, Felix. III. Senn, Hansjörg. IV. "Perioperative Chemotherapy" Symposium (1983 : Zurich University Hospital) V. Series: [DNLM: 1. Neoplasm Metastasis-prevention & control-congresses. 2. Neoplasms-drug therapy-congresses. 3. Neoplasms-surgery-congresses. 4. Postoperative Complications-prevention & control-congresses. RE106P v. 98 / QZ 267 P445 1983] RC261.R35 vol. 98 616.99'4 s 85-2747 [RC271.A35] [616.99'4061]

Softcover reprint of the hardcover 1st edition 1985

Typesetting: v. Starck'sche Druckereigesellschaft m.b.H., Wiesbaden
Binding: J. Schäffer OHG, Grünstadt

2125/3140-543210

Preface

One reason for failure to cure solid tumors by surgery appears to be the impossibility of controlling metastases that are present but latent at the time of operation. This failure is a common clinical experience with aggressive neoplasms, but it is not always appreciated in tumors with longer survival times, e. g., breast and colon cancer. In addition, recent evidence indicates that after resection of a primary tumor micrometastases from it might be enhanced by suppression of immune and reticuloendothelial functions of the host. Other factors, such as increase of coagulability and stress in the perioperative period, can also promote tumor growth. The development of new metastases might be facilitated by cells forced into the circulation during operative manipulations. Such events could be important for the outcome of treatment and it is suggested that preventive measures should be directed to this systemic component of solid tumors.
Radical surgery can reduce the number of tumor cells to a subclinical stage (10^3 to 10^6 cells) in which chemotherapy might be more effective than in advanced stages. Chemotherapy, on the other hand, might aggravate the surgical morbidity by influencing the wound healing process, by decreasing the immune response, and/or by toxicity to the bone marrow and to the gastrointestinal tract, for example.
In the continuous search for an optimal timing of surgery and chemotherapy in the multimodality approach to cancer, the disease-oriented Committees for Breast and Gastrointestinal Tumors of the Swiss Group for Clinical Cancer Research initiated the idea of a »Perioperative Chemotherapy« Symposium to be held at Zurich University Hospital. The aim was to collect basic research data and to update clinical experience with perioperative chemotherapy, to optimize the sequence of treatment modalities and to give surgeons and chemotherapists advice for future directions in both basic and clinical research in the combined effort in cancer therapy.
Very early in the organization of the Symposium it became evident that only a broad spectrum of international lecturers would assure achievement of the goals mentioned above. With the assistance of the Zurich

and Swiss Cancer League and some private institutions it was possible to arrange a meeting of some of the most competent and experienced people in the field of perioperative chemotherapy.
We have to express our thanks to those who presented papers at the Symposium, all acknowledged experts in their field, and to their colleagues who contributed to the published papers in this volume. We would also like to thank Dr. T. Thiekötter of Springer-Verlag for his advice and patient cooperation. Our thanks also go to Drs. D. Mona, C. Favez, and S. Youssef, and other members of the secretarial staff who helped in the excellent organization of the meeting in Zurich.
It seems that increasing numbers of surgeons throughout the world are prepared to subject their results to peer review and audit, and to accept the demanding discipline of multidisciplinary controlled trials. Such collaboration between surgical and medical oncologists will lead to steady improvements in the definitive management of patients with cancer. It is hoped that this publication may encourage further combined efforts in clinical cancer research.

Zurich and St. Gallen, Spring 1985

U. Metzger
F. Largiadèr
H.-J. Senn

Contents

*List of Contributors**

* The address of the principal author is given on the first page of each contribution
1 Page on which contribution begins

Frank M. Schabel, Jr. †

Director, Chemotherapy Research, Southern Research Institute,
Birmingham, USA

Frank M. Schabel, Jr. died suddenly and unexpectedly at the 13th International Cancer Congress in Vienna, on 30 August 1983. With his death we have lost one of the most brilliant and creative researchers in cancer treatment. His fundamental concepts developed in experimental cancer chemotherapy are well known all over the world. These concepts led directly to immediate, high-dose postoperative chemotherapy as an adjuvant to potentially curative surgery. There is no doubt that Frank M. Schabel's work initiated the idea of perioperative chemotherapy; hence, he might be called the father of perioperative adjuvant treatment of cancer. The editors of this volume are truly glad to start with the introduction given by Frank M. Schabel on the rationale of perioperative anticancer treatment, one of his last testimonies, which reflects his outstanding scientific ability, his intellectual integrity, and his talent for clarifying and solving the intricate problems of drug action in cancer.

The Editors

General Aspects

Rationale for Perioperative Anticancer Treatment

F. M. Schabel, Jr. †

Southern Research Institute, Birmingham, AL 35255, USA

I will limit my discussion essentially to chemotherapy as an adjuvant to surgery, since my experience is in this field, but I recognize that radiation therapy could be substituted for surgery in many cases and also that there are clinical examples of all three modalities being used in proper sequences with improved results over any two-modality treatment.
I would like to begin with a brief discussion of the need for perioperative chemotherapy.

Introduction

Figure 1 shows the number of cases of cancer that were metastatic at the time of clinical detection in the USA in 1977, the first year that approximately 1 million new cases of cancer occurred in the United States (DeVita et al. 1979). Since about 580,000 of these 1 million cases were cured by surgery and/or radiation treatment, DeVita stated that cancer had "the highest cure rate for any single category of chronic diseases in the United States" (DeVita et al. 1979).

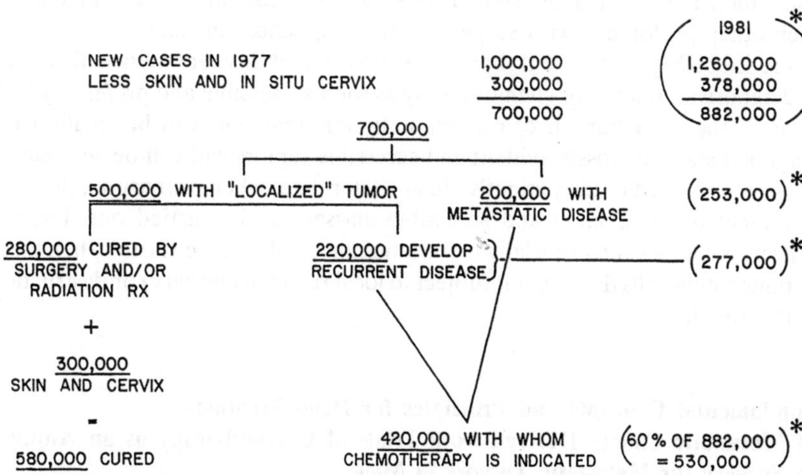

Fig. 1. Cancer in the United States of America. *Asterisk* indicates values estimated for 1981 from CA 31: 13 (1981)

This fact brought little comfort to most of the estimated 420,000 new patients with cancer in 1977 who could not be cured by surgery and/or radiation (the corresponding figure estimated for 1981 was 530,000). Chemotherapy, augmented with immunotherapy if available and useful, represents the only currently recognized hope of ultimate cure for cancer patients with metastatic disease at the time of diagnosis, since effective drugs are carried to most metastatic tumor sites by the blood or other body fluids. If drug treatment of these patients is delayed until the metastatic disease is clinically evident it usually fails because by that time the body burden of tumor stem cells exceeds the tumor cell kill potential of the best chemotherapy currently available. Obviously, we need better anticancer drugs, but since searches for new and better drugs are largely empirical, the time when these new and better drugs will be available cannot be predicted. Until they are discovered and developed, we need to use the available drugs more effectively. One clearly indicated approach is to use chemotherapy as an adjuvant to surgical treatment of tumors that are considered to be "localized" when they are first detected but are in fact systemic and recur later, often in metastatic sites far removed from the primary site (222,000 of 500,000 in the United States of America in 1977 and probably about 277,000 of 630,000 new cases with presumed localized tumors in 1981; Fig. 1). Cure rates with drug treatment of clinically evident systemic cancers have been low [11,000 cases cured (3%) of 420,000 cases in the United States in 1977] (DeVita et al. 1979), but the cure rate for systemic cancer is clearly rising and it has been estimated at about 40,000 per year in the United States at present (Silverberg 1981; DeVita et al. 1979). Of the more than 500,000 new patients each year in the United States of America who have systemic cancer at the time of diagnosis, those with presumed localized but actually systemic tumor that will recur after surgical removal or radiation treatment of the primary mass (estimated to have been about 277,000 cases in the USA in 1981; see Fig. 1) are the most likely to be cured with currently available drugs when these are used more effectively. Plausible interpretation of extensive data from trials of adjuvant chemotherapy with surgery against metastatic solid tumors of mice occurring in the major histological (organ and tissue) types of metastatic human cancer indicate some therapeutic principles that probably prevail in man. If data from animal models of human disease are relevant to the planning of treatment of similar diseases in man, then these principles should be seriously considered in the planning of adjuvant chemotherapy for use with surgery in treating cancer in man.

There is one logical course if there is a serious possibility that metastatic disease is present at diagnosis: initiation of chemotherapy as soon as possible and preferably before surgery, because the body burden of metastatic tumor stem cells will be smallest on the day of diagnosis and the grossly evident and accessible tumors will still be accessible and present no greater hazard to the patient's life at a later date, when primary surgical or radiological treatment of the evident and accessible masses can be carried out. Drug treatment of cancer, including and especially metastatic cancer, should be startet when the body burden of tumor stem cells that are not subject to local removal (surgery) or destruction (radiation) is the smallest.

Fundamental Concepts and Principles for Drug Treatment of Metastatic Cancer Derived from Trials of Chemotherapy as an Adjuvant to Surgery for Metastatic Tumors in Mice

Table 1 lists the fundamental concepts and basic principles that have been derived from extensive data obtained in trials of chemotherapy as an adjuvant to surgery in mice and

Table 1. Fundamental concepts and principles for drug treatment of metastatic cancer

Concept	Principle	Indication
1. Total body burden determines cure	First order kinetics of tumor cell kill by drugs	Treat when the total body burden is smallest
2. Population dynamics determines:		
A. Drug selection	Growth fraction is inversely related to population size	Drugs inactive against large tumors may be active against micrometastases
B. Treatment scheduling	Temporal phases of cell cycle and mass doubling time inversely related to size of individual metastases	Optimum drug treatment schedule changes as tumor cell number/metastasis decreases
3. Combination chemotherapy	Synergism for selective cytotoxicity and lack of cross-resistance	Use drug combinations lacking cross-resistance and less than additive in toxicity for vital normal cells

should be considered in planning curative adjuvant chemotherapy of metastatic cancer in man.

First-order kinetics of drug kill of tumor cells means that a constant percentage of tumor cells is killed by treatment with an effective drug, irrespective of the size of the tumor stem cell population, provided that (a) the population is metabolically homogeneous; and (b) for all tumor stem cells exposure to the drug(s) is equal in both concentration (C) and duration (time, T).

The basic principle clearly indicates that drug cure of systemic cancer in the adjuvant setting is dependent upon the body burden of tumor stem cells at the start of drug treatment.

Cancer chemotherapists have an advantage not usually available to antimicrobial chemotherapists, which is reduction of the body burden of tumor stem cells by surgical removal of grossly apparent and accessible tumor foci, thus reducing the total body burden of tumor stem cells to the range in which curative tumor cell kill can be achieved by the best available chemotherapy. This is the essence of adjuvant chemotherapy. Drug treatment of the recurrent disease, after initial surgical treatment of the primary tumor that was presumed to be localized at diagnosis and that did not show evidence of metastatic spread at the time of first surgical treatment, no longer has much chance of curing the condition, because of the large body burden, than does drug treatment of patients with grossly evident metastatic disease at the time of diagnosis. Cure rates in drug-treated patients with metastatic disease should be inversely related to the size and total number of metastases, and therefore, the earlier drug treatment of metastatic disease is started the higher the probability of cure. Adjuvant chemotherapy is therefore indicated as soon as possible after the surgical removal of grossly evident disease. In addition, since with few and limited exceptions effective anticancer drugs have steep dose-response curves, aggressive (high-dose) drug treatment is clearly indicated.

A large body of objective evidence from laboratory studies and subjective support from clinical trials indicate that small tumor foci (micrometastases) are more sensitive to chemotherapy than are large tumor foci. There are probably many reasons for this, including those discussed briefly here. (a) The growth fraction (GF)[1] of most tumors is inversely related to tumor mass, and it follows, therefore, that the smaller the tumor focus, the higher the fraction of proliferating tumor stem cells in each micrometastatic site. The tumor cells in the GF are more sensitive to drug kill by all classes of drugs. (b) A greater blood supply in small than in large tumor foci will allow more uniform exposure of cells to cytotoxic drug levels. (c) The cell division cycle time (Tc) of tumor stem cells has been shown to be related to the size of the tumor focus – the larger the tumor focus, the longer the Tc of the tumor cells. These circumstances are directly relevant to drug selection and optimum treatment schedule for greatest drug kill of tumor stem cells at metastatic tumor sites, especially in the adjuvant setting, where large numbers of inapparent micrometastases may be present (Schabel 1975; Schabel and Simpson-Herren, to be published). Since the total body burden of tumor stem cells that must be killed to achieve cure, even in the adjuvant chemotherapy setting after tumor reduction by surgery, is unknown but may be, and probably often is, large, combination chemotherapy is indicated. The selection of drugs for use in adjuvant chemotherapy should be directed at the same therapeutic benefits as are sought in the selection of drugs for treatment of more advanced and grossly evident disease, (a) greater selective cytotoxicity for tumor cells; (b) less-than-additive toxicity for vital normal cells than any of the components (one or more) of the drug combination; and (c) cytotoxic activity of one or more of the components of the drug combination for tumor stem cells in the body burden of the metastatic disease that are resistant to one or more of the other drugs in the drug combination. This is a particularly important aspect of drug selection for any drug treatment regimen, and the probability that drug-resistant tumor cells are present is directly related to the body burden of tumor stem cells at the start of drug treatment.

Chemotherapy of Metastatic Solid Tumors of Mice as an Adjuvant to Surgery

Examples of improved cure rates obtained at the Southern Research Institute with chemotherapy as an adjuvant to surgery and illustrating the principles and concepts listed in Table 1 are shown in Figs. 2–5.

Lewis Lung Carcinoma

The Lewis lung carcinoma (Fig. 2) arose spontaneously in 1951 as a carcinoma of the lung in a C57BL mouse and has been maintained in continuous serial passage. It is a highly anaplastic type of epidermoid carcinoma. It metastasizes, primarily to the lungs, very soon after subcutaneous implantation and leads to death from massive tumor growth in the lungs. Surgical removal of the primary tumor after metastatic spread to the lungs does not increase the life-span.

1 The growth fraction is the fraction of the total tumor stem cell population that is in the active cell division cycle at any given time

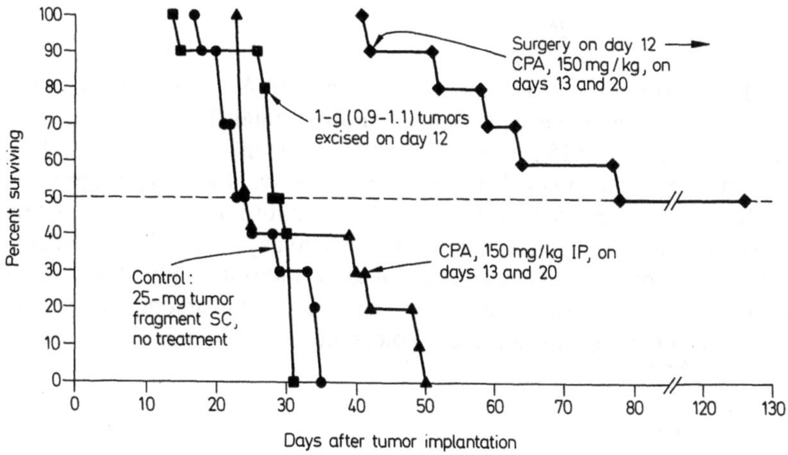

Fig. 2. Survival of BDF_1 mice following implantation of Lewis lung carcinoma treated by surgery and adjuvant chemotherapy

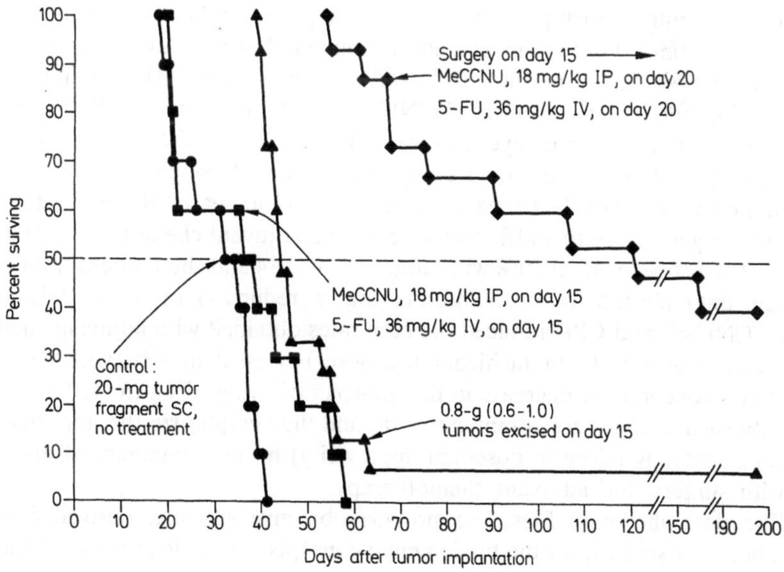

Fig. 3. Survival of BALB/C mice following implantation of colon tumor line 26 treated by surgery and adjuvant chemotherapy

Surgical removal of the primary tumor on day 12 after implantation or treatment with cyclophosphamide (CPA) on days 13 and 20 after implantation failed either to cure mice or to extend their life-span significantly. However, surgical removal of the primary tumor on day 12 and CPA treatment on days 13 and 20 resulted in a significant increase in the life-span of animals ultimately dying of tumor.

Colon Tumor Line 26

The line 26 colon tumor is a metastatic, *N*-nitroso-*N*-methylurethane-induced transplantable colon tumor of mice, which is uniformly fatal if untreated (Corbett et al. 1975). Surgery alone on day 15 cured less than 10% of the mice, and MeCCNU + 5-FU on day 15 without surgery had no evident therapeutic activity. However, surgery on day 15 followed by MeCCNU + 5-FU 5 days later (day 20) cured 40% of the mice and extended the median life-span of animals dying of tumor by about 30 days beyond the median of those treated with surgery only. These results are of great interest, since MeCCNU + 5-FU, with or without added vincristine, has been reported to be among the best drug treatments observed to date against advanced colorectal cancer and gastric cancer in man (Moertel 1975).

C3H Mammary Adenocarcinoma Line 44

The C3H mammary adenocarcinoma was established by transplantation from a spontaneous mammary carinoma in a C3H/HeN mouse, and its metastatic potential was increased by selective subcutaneous transplantation of naturally occurring metastatic foci from the lungs, which produced a highly anaplastic and metastatic tumor (Schabel 1976). Surgical removal of the subcutaneously implanted primary tumor on day 11 to day 14 after implantation failed to cure 70%–90% of mice (Fig. 4). Treatment with *N*,*N'*-bis (2-chloroethyl)-*N*-nitrosourea (BCNU) + CPA or with *cis*-4 [[[(2-chloroethyl)nitroso-amino]carboamyl]amino]cyclohexane carboxylic acid (CCCNU-*cis*) + CPA on days 15–18 after implantation failed to cure any of the mice. However, BCNU + CPA 4 days after surgical removal of the primary tumor on day 11 increased the cure rate from about 30% with surgery alone to 100% with surgery and adjuvant chemotherapy (Fig. 4A) and from less than 10% to about 50% with surgery on day 14 and chemotherapy on day 18 (Fig. 4B). The data plotted in Fig. 5 indicate that a reduction of about 33% in the doses of CCCNU-*cis* and CPA reduced the cure rates obtained with adjuvant chemotherapy from greater than 80% (with the higher drug doses) to less than 50% (with the lower drug doses) with a concomitant decrease in the life-span of dying, drug-treated mice. Dose-response data such as these are commonly seen, and they emphasize the importance of aggressive chemotherapy (close to dose-limiting toxicity) in the attainment of maximum cure rates with surgery and adjuvant chemotherapy.

The data shown in Figs. 2–5 provide objective support, derived from a number of laboratory studies, for the fundamental concepts and basic principles (Table 1) relating to curative adjuvant chemotherapy with a number of solid tumors of mice following surgical removal of the primary tumor after metastasis has occurred. The data in Fig. 6 illustrate that: (a) The incidence of metastatic spread from the primary tumor site and the size of the body burden of metastatic tumor stem cells are directly related to the size of the primary tumor mass, although there is great variability in the numbers of metastatic tumor stem cells with primary tumors that are quite similar in size. In this regard, these metastatic tumors of mice appear to be quite similar to primary breast cancers in women (Fig. 4). (b) Cure rates with effective drugs as adjuvant treatment to surgery are directly related to the primary tumor mass at the time of surgery (Fig. 4) and the dose of the effective drug used (Fig. 5). (c) Noncurative response of a grossly apparent primary tumor to any drug indicates the use of that drug (or another of the same functional or kinetic activity class, e.g., cell-cycle-specific or cell-cycle-nonspecific) for postsurgical treatment of likely

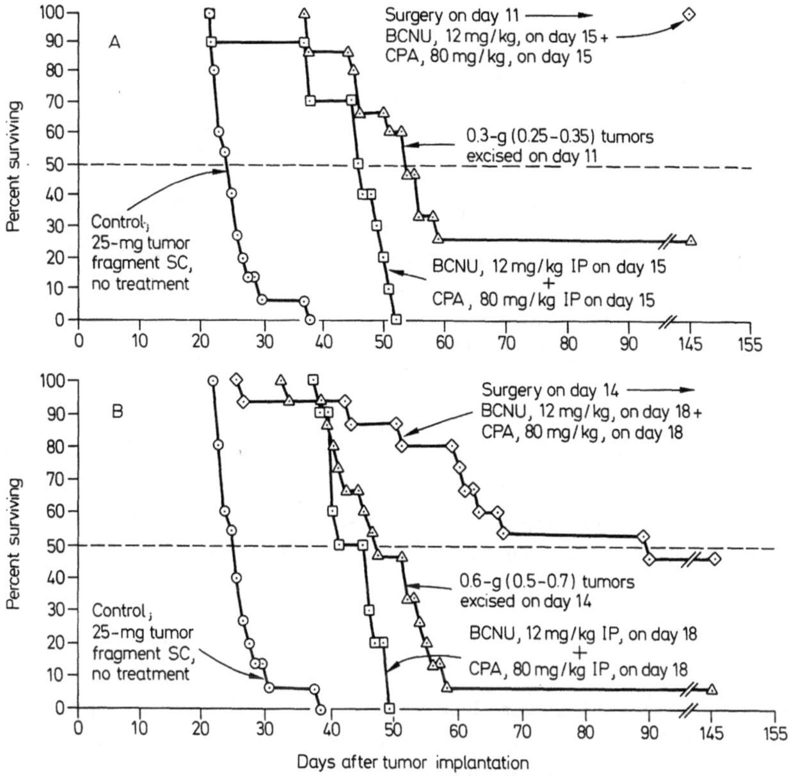

Fig. 4 A, B. Survival of B_6C3F_1 mice with C3H mammary tumor line 44 treated by **A** surgery on day 11 and chemotherapy on day 15 or **B** surgery on day 14 and chemotherapy on day 18

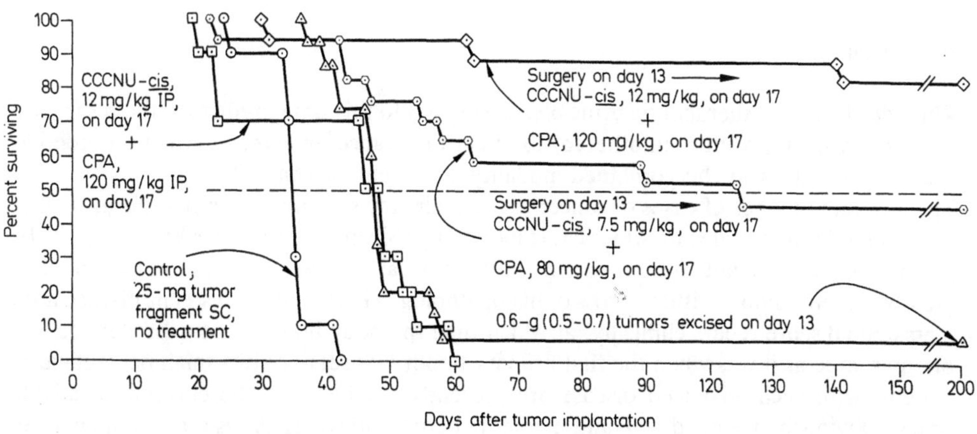

Fig. 5. Survival of B_6C3F_1 mice with C3H mammary tumor line 44 treated by surgery and chemotherapy at various dosages

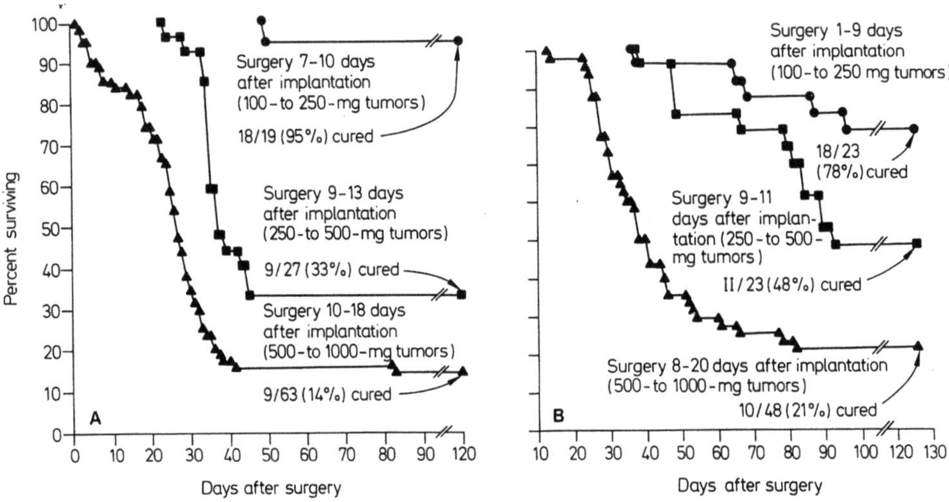

Fig. 6 A, B. Cumulative mortality from metastatic disease after surgical removal of progressively staged primary tumors. **A** Mammary adenocarcinoma line 44 in C3H mice; **B** colon carcinoma line 26 in BALB/C mice

micrometastases. However, lack of response of the grossly apparent tumor to any anticancer drug should not exclude it from consideration for use in the treatment of micrometastases as an adjuvant to surgery. It has repeatedly been shown that drugs with no apparent useful therapeutic activity against a large body burden of tumor stem cells consisting of the primary tumor and micrometastases were able to cure varying but significant numbers of animals when used as adjuvant chemotherapy in conjunction with surgical treatment.

Discussion

What do the chemotherapeutic principles developed to this time predict for the future use of surgery with adjuvant chemotherapy for metastatic cancer in man, and what is needed to speed up progress in the combined-modality treatment of cancer?

The absolute number of cases of cancer that are already systemic when first diagnosed, at least in the United States of America, is increasing (Silverberg 1975; DeVita et al. 1979). Physicians are reluctant to treat patients after surgical removal or radiation treatment of grossly evident tumors without gross or histopathological evidence of systemic disease until metastatic disease recurs clinically, at which time the body burden of tumor stem cells is often as large as it was when the first primary tumor was seen; only a small percentage of patients with such advanced disease are presently curable with the currently available drugs. Obviously, we need new and markedly better anticancer drugs than we now have. Since the time when these new drugs will be available cannot be predicted, improvement of the cure rate in systemic cancer by more effective use of the currently available drugs must be attempted.

All scientific principles relating to effective (curative) chemotherapy of cancer and experience to date clearly indicate that cure rates with anticancer drugs are directly related to the body burden of tumor stem cells at the start of therapy and that the cure rates that can be attained with chemotherapy are directly related to adequate drug doses. This being the case, drug treatment with curative intent should be started *as early as possible* and treatment should be aggressive (high dose). Unless objective evidence of the presence of potentially life-threatening micrometastatic disease is present at the time of surgical removal of the primary tumor, treatment of all patients with aggressive chemotherapy exposes all of them to a similar risk of toxic side-effects of the drug therapy, including those with no residual tumor stem cells and hence no risk of recurrence. This is considered a minimal risk if the probability of recurrent metastatic disease is high, e.g., 80% of osteosarcoma patients and 85% of women with breast cancer and four histologically positive lymph nodes (Fig. 7). Withholding adjuvant chemotherapy from women subjected to surgery for breast cancer who have no evidence of metastatic spread (histologically negative lymph nodes) at the time of surgical resection of the primary tumor and axillary node dissection but whose disease later recurs (25% of patients) is an unacceptable risk to these patients, because early postsurgical chemotherapy, particularly if aggressive, would probably cure most of them.

In my judgment, the greatest limitation to improving cancer chemotherapy of both clinically evident disease and clinically unrecognized early primary or micrometastatic disease is the lack of sensitive markers for tumor stem cells in some available source such as plasma, lymph, urine, or other body fluids of humans and animals bearing life-threatening malignant neoplasms.

If adequate markers for tumor stem cells were available, we could:

1. Estimate the body burden of tumor stem cells. If this were possible we would no longer treat the 15% of women with breast cancer and four positive axillary lymph nodes after mastectomy who do not have recurrence of their clinical evident disease or the 20% of osteosarcoma patients cured by surgical removal of the primary tumor. Of far greater importance, we would treat and probably would not lose the 25% of women with systemic breast cancer but with negative lymph nodes draining the primary tumor, who

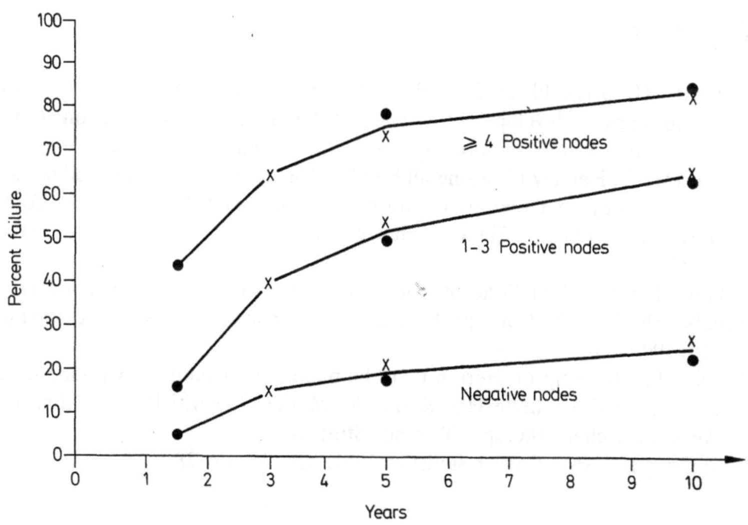

Fig. 7. Treatment failures after radical mastectomy. ●, data from NSABP, USA (1975); ×, data from Milan, Italy (1978)

currently do not receive adjuvant chemotherapy following surgery because only one in four of these patients is at risk of recurrence.

2. If tumor stem cells were present and drug treatment was used, with adequate markers we could determine drug sensitivity and the net change in body burden of tumor stem cells caused by treatment. If no net reduction of tumor stem cells was caused by drug treatment we should know that either the drugs being used were inactive or they were not being used in an optimum dose or the schedule was not ideal.
3. If the body burden of tumor stem cells was reduced but resumed growth under initially cytotoxic drug treatment, the overgrowth of drug-resistant tumor stem cells would be likely and a change of treatment to other drugs would be clearly indicated.
4. Finally, and of great importance, cancer chemotherapists would be able to know when the body burden of life-threatening tumor stem cells was below the number capable of re-establishing the clinically evident disease. At that point, drug treatment could be terminated and cure could be assumed with confidence. Until that utopian day, drug treatment of metastatic cancer, particularly as an adjuvant to surgery, will be best guided by the principles indicated by adjuvant chemotherapy of metastatic murine tumors: (a) Begin treatment as soon as possible after surgical removal of the primary tumor; and (b) treat aggressively (high dose, short duration) with the drug(s) with the greatest probable selective cytotoxicity for tumor cells over vital normal cells according to all available practical experience combined with such information on biochemical and tumor growth kinetics as can be obatined.

My closing thought is this:
If drug treatment is not considered without the demonstrated presence of metastatic disease, which means, for example, that adjuvant chemotherapy is not considered after surgery in breast patients with negative axillary nodes, then real progress must await the discovery and development of reliable and sensitive tumor stem cell markers. Without such markers, adjuvant chemotherapy following primary surgery or radiation for clinically inapparent micrometastases in man or animals will remain subjective and empirical.

References

Corbett TH, Griswold DP Jr, Roberts BT, Peckham JC, Schabel FM Jr (1975) Tumor induction relationships in development of transplantable cancers of the colon in mice for chemotherapy assays, with a note on carcinogen structure. Cancer Res 35: 2434–2439

DeVita VT Jr, Henney JE, Stonehill E (1979) Cancer mortality: the good news. In: Jones SE, Salmon SE (eds) Adjuvant therapy of cancer II. Grune and Stratton, New York, pp XV–XX

Moertel CG (1975) Clinical management of advanced gastrointestinal cancer. Cancer 36: 675–682

Schabel FM Jr (1975) Concepts for systemic treatment of micrometastases. Cancer 35: 15–24

Schabel FM Jr (1976) Concepts for treatment of micrometastases developed in murine systems. AJl 126: 500–511

Schabel FM Jr, Simpson-Herren L (to be published) Tumor growth kinetics and drug treatment of cancer. In: Kuemmerle HP, Karrer K, Mathé G, Periti P (eds) Clinical chemotherapy, vol 3. Anticancer chemotherapy. Thieme, Stuttgart

Silverberg E (1981) Cancer statistics 1981. CA 31: 13–28

*Surgical Intervention and Metastasis**

R. Keller

Institut für Immunologie und Virologie, Universität Zürich, Arbeitsgruppe für Immunbiologie, Schönleinstrasse 22, 8032 Zürich, Switzerland

Introduction

It is now appreciated that the tumor-host relationship is intimate and complex, and that the outcome of tumor disease depends on many variables pertaining to both host and tumor. This implies that each tumor-host relationship has individual features; accordingly, there are few valid general conclusions to be drawn from the immense effort focused on this problem. Despite these reservations it is possible to identify certain major issues that are applicable in a variety of clinical and experimental situations. As some of these issues may well be relevant to the establishment of more appropriate therapeutic regimens they are briefly outlined here. The experimental examples were derived from the D-12 rat fibrosarcoma, a model studied extensively in this laboratory (Keller 1980, 1981, to be published).

Systemic Nature of Most Malignancies

There is now broad consensus that most cancer treatment failures are attributable not to the locally growing primary tumor but rather to the host's inability to control its spread and establishment at secondary sites (Roos and Dingemans 1980; Sugarbaker and Ketcham 1977; Weiss 1977; Willis 1973). This observation is valid for "liquid" cancers (leukemia, many lymphomas); for highly malignant neoplasms such as those of the lung, pancreas or stomach; and, remarkably enough, also for tumors with lower degrees of malignancy. The fact is that tumors which clinically appear to be localized are often on the way to becoming systemic by the time the primary tumor is diagnosed. Our new ability to achieve relatively early detection of established secondary tumor cell foci has led to a realistic awareness of the scope of this problem. Accordingly, it now seems evident that in varied clinical and experimental situations the dissemination of tumor cells is an early event and is a process that continues.

* This work was supported by the Swiss National Science Foundation (grants 3.173.77 and 3.609.80) and the Canton of Zurich

Recent Results in Cancer Research. Vol. 98

Phenotypic Heterogeneity of Disseminated Tumor Cells

It has been known for some time that the cell populations found in a malignant tumor are heterogeneous, but it is only recently that attention has been directed to specific aspects such as their growth behavior and metastatic properties, their biochemical characteristics, and most compellingly, to their immunogenic attributes and their susceptibility to various modes of therapeutic intervention. These studies have revealed wide variations in the metastatic potential of subpopulations from the same tumor (Weiss 1979; Hart and Fidler 1981; Nicolson 1982; Poste 1982; Fig. 1). It is likely that such variants arise as a consequence either of genetic variability or of the subjection of such cell populations to various host selection pressures (immunoselection). Heterogeneity as regards metastatic capability implies that different metastases derived from the same tumor could yield cells differing in their metastatic potential. In malignant cancers that carry a high risk of early metastasis, tumor cells with a high metastatic potential are assuredly present at a very early stage in the emergence of the primary neoplasm. However, it remains controversial whether metastasis reflects stable cells of a pre-existing phenotype and is a predetermined, nonrandom event (Fidler and Kripke 1977) or whether many, if not all, cancer cells have inherent metastatic potential and are recruited randomly (Weiss 1979).

Efficiency of the Metastatic Process: Generally Low

Clinical and experimental evidence suggests that the detachment of viable tumor cells from the primary tumor is a spontaneous and continuing process (Butler and Gullino 1975; Kleinerman and Liotta 1977; Sugarbaker 1979; Roos and Dingemans 1980). There is often a close correlation between the size of the primary tumor and the incidence of histologically verified metastasis (Fig. 2). It is noteworthy, however, that even very small primary tumors, e.g., breast cancers (Sugarbaker et al. 1982), can occasionally develop metastases. During progressive tumor growth the number of neoplastic cells entering the circulation is rather large. Although tumors metastasize via both the blood and the lymphatic

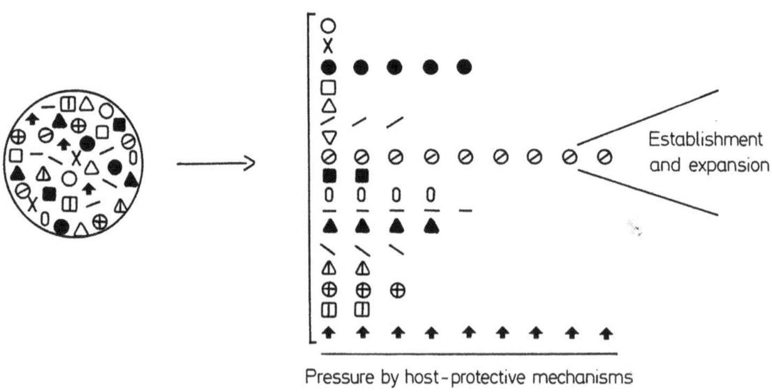

Fig. 1. Primary tumor cells are heterogeneous; only a few tumor cells are able to adapt and survive. Two major concepts have been used to account for the metastatic inefficiency of tumor cells: (a) stable, pre-existing metastatic phenotype, according to which metastasis and metastatic inefficiency result from nonrandom processes; and (b) inherent metastatic potential of many cells, according to which metastasis and metastatic inefficiency are basically random events

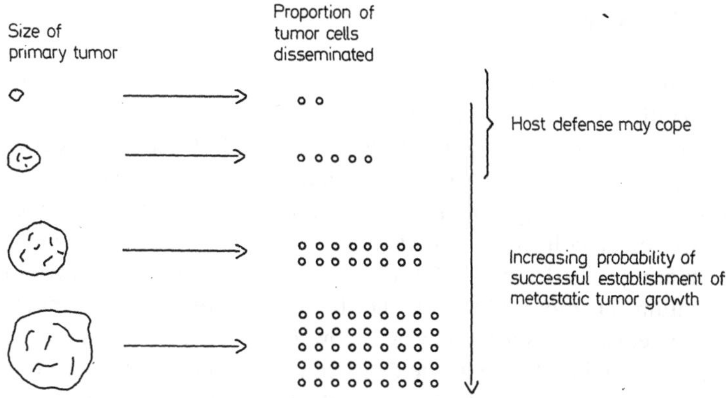

Fig. 2. Relationship between size of primary tumor and tumor cell dissemination. The host may cope with tumor cells when only a few cells are disseminated per unit of time; as the number of disseminated tumor cells increases so does the probability of establishment of metastatic tumor growth

Fig. 3. Localization of primary tumor and incidence of spontaneous and induced lymph node metastases in the D-12 rat fibrosarcoma system. *C*, percent incidence of spontaneous metastases. In localization *1*, the proportion of spontaneous macroscopic metastases remained at ≤ 10% irrespective of the size of th primary tumor implant. In localization *2*, the incidence of spontaneous macroscopic metastases was around 15% until the local tumor had reached a size of approximately 10 mm but then increased with increasing tumor size. Surgical intervention, performed when the primary tumor inoculum had reached a size of 5–8 mm [in localization *1* surgical excision (*SE*); in localization *2* amputation of the thigh (*A*)], was followed in a considerable proportion of the animals by rapid outgrowth of macroscopic metastases, which also emerged in more distant lymph nodes

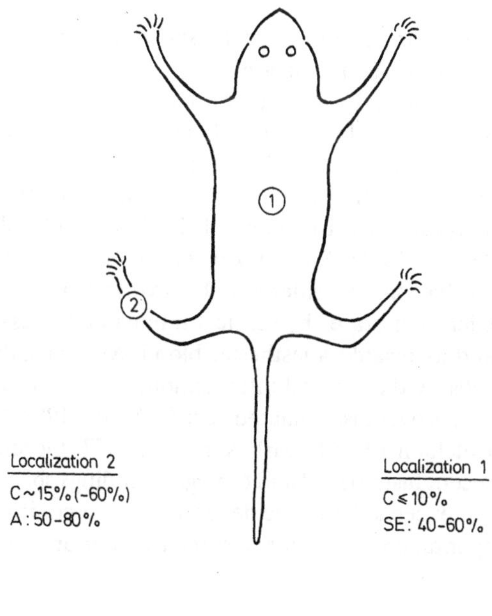

circulation, carcinomas more frequently metastasize to regional lymph nodes at a comparatively early stage in their development, whereas sarcomas spread more readily via the hematogenous route. Studies in experimental systems have shown that the bulk of tumor cells that are blood borne do not survive circulation (Fidler 1976, 1978); other clinical and experimental evidence, although less extensive, suggests that the lymph nodes may constitute an equally hostile environment (Kurokawa 1970; Kodama 1977; Carr and Carr 1980; Mitchell 1980; Weiss 1980). Consequently, it is only the relatively few tumor cells capable of surviving the adverse conditions in the circulation and in tissues and of escaping from local host defenses that are likely to succeed in establishing metastatic tumor growth.

Localization of Metastases

The site of the primary tumor and its relation to the peripheral circulation and/or the lymphatics are important in determining the localization of metastases. However, the high frequency of nonrandom dissemination of neoplastic cells into certain organs suggests that various other factors, such as the innate properties of circulating tumor cells and their products, especially membrane fragments, host capillary endothelium, and organ environment, collectively dictate tumor cell fate in vivo rather than the mere distribution of circulating cells. In the D-12 rat fibrosarcoma model, progressive local growth of a tumor inoculum in the middle of the back was followed by macroscopically detectable spontaneous metastases only in a low proportion of the animals; in contrast, primary implantation into the thigh yielded frequent spontaneous macroscopic metastases (Fig. 3). As the number of invading tumor cells per node is smaller in situations where draining involves more than a single lymph node, the rate at which tumor cells enter the regional lymph nodes may well be a determining factor.

Postulated Versus Established Consequences of Surgery

The aforementioned data show that in humans and in many experimental systems metastasis is a function of tumor size and the rate of tumor growth. Whether surgical resection of the local tumor results in cure or in systemic recurrence is largely dependent on whether viable tumor cells were already present in the circulation and/or had reached distant organs (Table 1). Once viable tumor cells have established growth at distant sites, excision of the primary tumor can be followed promptly by accelerated progression of metastatic disease (Tyzzer 1913; Lewis and Cole 1958; Schatten 1958; Ketcham et al. 1961; Kinsey 1961; Sugarbaker et al. 1977; Keller 1981; Fig. 3). Among the biological mechanisms considered to be involved are the possible stimulation of established systemic micrometastases by surgical trauma and stress, the immunosuppressive effects of surgery and associated anesthesia, blood hypercoagulability, mechanical dissemination of tumor cells by the surgical intervention, and loss of the inhibitory effect that the primary tumor exerts over disseminated cells (Schatten 1958; Simpson-Herren et al. 1976; Sugarbaker and Ketcham 1977; Sugarbaker et al. 1977; Gorelik 1982). In the D-12 fibrosarcoma system, recent histological and biological findings showing that the incidence of micrometastases by far exceeded the incidence of macroscopically evident metastases have indicated that spontaneous secondary spread of tumor cells had already taken place prior to surgery

Table 1. Possible consequences of surgical removal of primary tumor

	Neoplastic cells in other tissues		Expected consequence of surgical intervention
Established local primary tumor	None	⟶	Cure
	A few micrometastases	⟶	Cure, dormancy and/or outgrowth of metastases
	Micro- and macrometastases	⟶	Outgrowth of metastases

(Keller and Hess 1982). Accordingly, it is postulated that surgical removal of the primary tumor enhances the outgrowth of already established micrometastases rather than inducing the spread of neoplastic cells. Further experiments based on various kinds of surgical intervention have shown that control hind limb amputation had no effect on the frequency, size, or localization of metastases; in contrast, equivalent amputation of the tumor-bearing limb resulted in a marked increase in the incidence of macroscopic metastases, which also developed in more locations. Accordingly, surgical intervention and the changes associated with it do not themselves seem to constitute a major component in the promotion of secondary tumor growth in this particular model (Keller, to be published).

In conclusion, present knowledge indicates that (a) most malignancies are already on the way to becoming systemic at the time they are diagnosed; and (b) surgical removal of the primary tumor may give rise to rapid outgrowth of pre-existing micrometastases. Consequently, even in the absence of clinically detectable secondaries, surgical intervention should no longer represent the only means of treatment for local primary neoplasia. Combination with other adequate adjuvant regimens is imperative. It is hoped that our increasing understanding of the biology of experimental metastasis will result in a progressive resolution of this major clinical problem.

Summary

Recent findings, briefly summarized here, show that the dissemination of neoplastic cells is an early and continuing process; that individual tumor cells in a malignant tumor possess differing metastatic capacities; and that metastases can arise from specific subpopulations of tumor cells. These findings have considerable implications for the understanding and treatment of systemic malignancies. The underlying cause for the finding that surgical removal of the primary local tumor is often followed by considerably enhanced outgrowth of established micrometastases is not yet understood. The trauma and stress associated with surgical intervention does not of itself seem to constitute a *major* tumor-promoting component. More likely candidates responsible for enhanced outgrowth of metastases after surgery are the removal of the growth-inhibitory restraint that the primary tumor exerts on disseminated neoplastic cells.

References

Butler TP, Gullino PM (1975) Qantitation of cell shedding into efferent blood of mammary adenocarcinoma. Cancer Res 35: 512–516

Carr I, Carr J (1980) Experimental lymphatic invasion and metastasis. In: Weiss L, Gilbert HA, Ballon SC (eds) Lymphatic system metastasis. Hall, Boston, pp 41–73

Fidler IJ (1976) Patterns of tumor cell arrest and development. In: Weiss L (ed) Fundamental aspects of metastasis. North-Holland, Amsterdam, pp 275–289

Fidler IJ (1978) General considerations for studies of experimental cancer metastasis. Methods Cancer Res 15: 399–439

Fidler IJ, Kripke ML (1977) Metastasis results from pre-existing variant cells within a malignant tumor. Science 197: 893–895

Gorelik E (1982) Antimetastatic concomitant immunity. In: Liotta LA, Hart IR (eds) Tumor invasion and metastasis. Nijhoff, The Hague, pp 113–131

Hart IR, Fidler IJ (1981) The implication of tumor heterogeneity for studies in the biology and therapy of cancer metastasis. Biochim Biophys Acta 651: 37–50

Keller R (1980) Distinctive characteristics of host tumor resistance in a rat fibrosarcoma model system. In: van Furth R (ed) Mononuclear phagocytes. Functional aspects. Nijhoff, The Hague, pp 1725–1740
Keller R (1981) Induction of macroscopic metastases via surgery. The site of the primary tumor inoculum is critical. Invasion and Metastasis 1: 136–148
Keller R (to be published) Elicitation of macroscopic metastases via surgery: various forms of surgical intervention differ in their induction of metastatic outgrowth
Keller R, Hess MW (1982) Divergency between incidence of microscopic and macroscopic metastases. Virchows Arch A 398: 33–43
Ketcham AS, Kinsey DL, Wexler H, Mantel N (1961) The development of spontaneous metastases after the removal of the primary tumor. Cancer 14: 875–881
Kinsey DL (1961) Effects of surgery upon cancer metastasis. JAMA 178: 734–735
Kleinerman J, Liotta L (1977) Release of tumor cells. In: Day SB, Stansly P, Laird Myers SP, Garattini S, Lewis MG (eds) Cancer invasion and metastasis: biologic mechanisms and therapy. Raven, New York, pp 135–143
Kodama T (1977) Pathology of immunologic regression of tumor metastases in the lymph nodes. Gann Monogr Cancer Res 20: 83–91
Kurokawa Y (1970) Experiments on lymph node metastasis by intralymphatic inoculation of rat ascites tumor cells, with special reference to lodgement, passage, and growth of tumor cells in lymph nodes. Gan 61: 461–471
Lewis MR, Cole WH (1958) Experimental increase in lung metastases after operative trauma. Arch Surg 77: 621–626
Mitchell MS (1980) A note on the lymph node as an immunologic barrier. In: Weiss L, Gilbert HA, Ballon SC (eds) Lymphatic system metastasis. Hall, Boston, pp 74–79
Nicolson GL (1982) Cancer metastasis: organ colonization and the cell surface properties of malignant cells. Biochim Biophys Acta 695: 113–176
Poste G (1982) Experimental systems for analysis of the malignant phenotype. Cancer Metast Rev 1: 141–199
Roos R, Dingemans KP (1980) Mechanisms of metastasis. Biochim Biophys Acta 650: 135–166
Schatten WE (1958) An experimental study of postoperative tumor metastases. I. Growth of pulmonary metastases following total removal of primary leg tumor. Cancer 11: 455–459
Simpson-Herren L, Sanford AH, Holmquist JP (1976) Effects of surgery on the cell kinetics of residual tumor. Cancer Treat Rep 60: 1749–1760
Sugarbaker EV (1979) Cancer metastasis: a product of tumor-host interactions. Curr Probl Cancer 7: 1–59
Sugarbaker EV, Ketcham A (1977) Mechanisms and prevention of cancer dissemination: an overview. Semin Oncol 4: 19–32
Sugarbaker EV, Thornthwaite J, Ketcham AS (1977) Inhibitory effect of a primary tumor on metastasis. In: Day SB, Stansly P, Laird Myers WP, Garattini S, Lewis MG (eds) Cancer invasion and metastasis: biologic mechanisms and therapy. Raven, New York, pp 227–240
Sugarbaker EV, Weingrad DN, Roseman JM (1982) Observations on cancer metastasis in man. In: Liotta LA, Hart IR (eds) Tumor invasion and metastasis. Nijhoff, The Hague, pp 427–465
Tyzzer EE (1913) Factors in the production and growth of tumor metastases. J Med Res 28: 309–312
Weiss L (1977) A pathologic overview of metastasis. Semin Oncol 4: 5–17
Weiss L (1979) Dynamic aspects of cancer cell populations in metastasis. Am J Pathol 97: 601–608
Weiss L (1980) The pathophysiology of metastasis within the lymphatic system. In: Weiss L, Gilbert HA, Ballon SC (eds) Lymphatic system metastasis. Hall, Boston, pp 2–40
Willis RA (1973) The spread of tumours in the human body, 3rd edn. Butterworths, London

Effect of Chemotherapy and Radiotherapy on Wound Healing: Experimental Studies

R. Shamberger

The Children's Hospital, 300 Longwood Avenue, Boston, MA 02115, USA

Introduction

Perioperative chemotherapy is increasing in use and importance, as is indicated by the very fact of this conference. Its use is designed to achieve cure in a larger number of patients than can be cured by surgery alone. Patients now receive chemotherapy or radiotherapy either before surgical resection, to improve the results of standard treatment or to increase the possibility of removal of large lesions, or following surgery, to remove any microscopic remnants of tumor following resection.

Over the last two decades experimental data have suggested that antineoplastic agents are most effective when the tumor burden is low. More recent clinical studies of adjuvant chemotherapy have supported this finding. Administration of perioperative antineoplastic agents, whether in this adjuvant setting or to decrease tumor bulk prior to resection, must be weighed against the risks to the patient. One of the major concerns regarding these agents is the effect they will produce on primary wound healing. The purpose of this report is to review the experimental studies of antineoplastic agents and radiotherapy on wound healing. A basic understanding of the wound healing process and the effect of antineoplastic agents and radiotherapy on it will allow perioperative treatment plans to be designed with minimum risks to the patient. Consideration must be given to the time interval between administration of the agents and surgery as well as to the agents employed.

The Wound Healing Process and Its Assessment

Edward Howes in 1929 provided the basis for study of the incised wound (Howes et al. 1929). He correlated the histological stages of healing with the gain in tensile strength confirmed by later authors (Levenson et al. 1965). The early phase of healing (days 1–6), which he termed the "latent phase," was characterized by an active infiltration of the fibrin coagulum with polymorphonuclear neutrophils (PMN), macrophages, and fibroblasts, followed by vascular infiltration. This is clearly a period of active cellular migration and metabolism and should be more accurately termed the "proliferative phase" (Fig. 1). The wound has minimal tensile strength at this stage. The second phase of healing is the "maturation" or "collagen phase," in which there is active synthesis of collagen and fibroblast proliferation. It is associated with a rapid gain in tensile strength. Although the

Recent Results in Cancer Research. Vol. 98

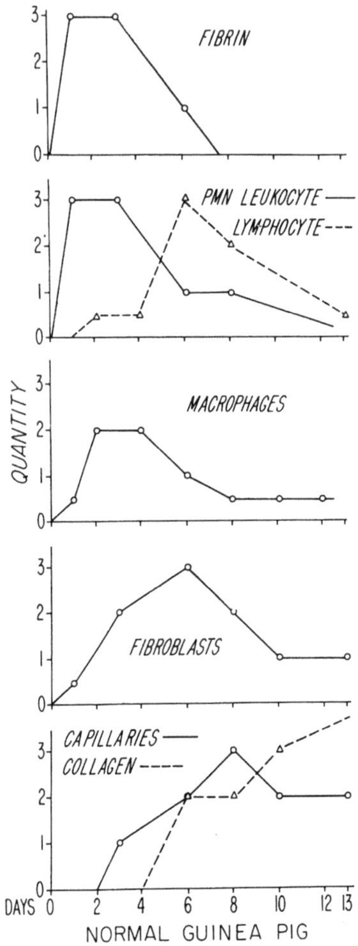

Fig. 1. Schematic showing the content and progression of cellular infiltration of an incised wound. Early appearance of fibrin, leukocytes, and macrophages is shown, with later appearance of fibroblasts, capillaries and collagen. Estimates shown are derived from the number of cells or elements per high-power field as seen in five sections of each wound. (Adapted from Ross and Benditt 1962)

healing of an incised wound is a continuous process, most subsequent authors have divided it into similar stages, as shown in Fig. 2.

The primary closed wound is used most frequently to study the effect of chemotherapeutic agents. It is the most clinically applicable model and the most readily quantitated. Several specific wounds have been studied, including gastric, small bowel, colonic, laparotomy (musculofascial), and dermal wounds. Each wound has specific benefits as well as limitations (Table 1). Levenson and colleagues argue strongly that laparotomy wounds are too complex to provide consistent results and favor a dermal wound model (Levenson et al. 1964). Other authors feel the musculofascial laparotomy wound is the most clinically relevant (Desprez and Kien 1960; Farhat et al. 1958, 1959; Gupta et al. 1970. Hardesty 1958; Morris et al. 1978). Studies of open granulating wounds are less clinically applicable and it is more difficult to quantitate the rate of healing in these. They are also more subject to "environmental" variables than are the incised and primarily closed wounds.

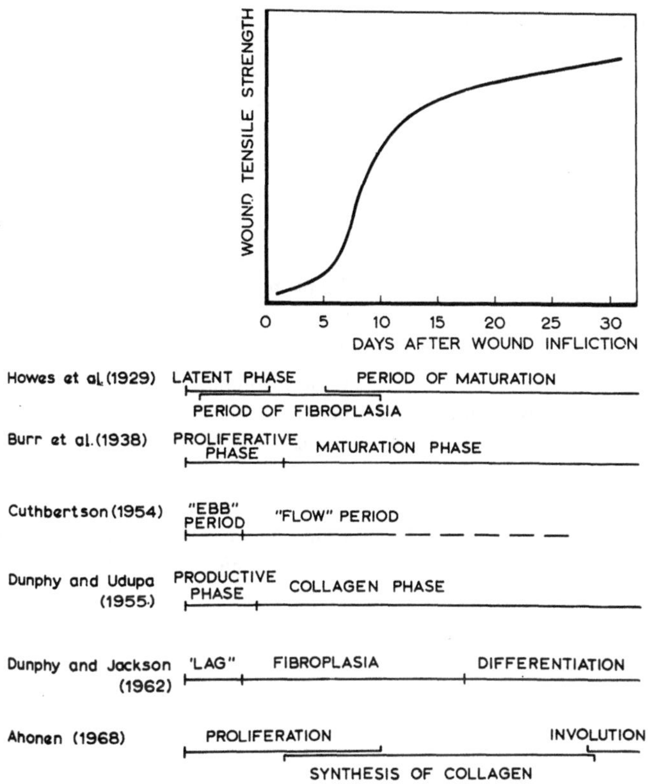

Fig. 2. Schematic showing the time course of the rise in wound tensile strength and the large number of terms given by various authors to the phases of healing. (Niinikoski 1969)

Measurement of Tensile Strength

The methods used in measurement of wound strength must be assessed for their reliability. Enteric wounds are often tested by distension of the viscus with air or fluid with measurement of the "rupture pressure." This method is subject to error because the tension in the wound (T) is related not only to the pressure (P) but also to the radius (R) of the organ according to the law of Laplace ($T = P X R$). This relationship of tension to pressure is frequently ignored. Any variable that will decrease the thickness of the viscus wall, such as starvation, and thus increase its radius at a given pressure will have a significant effect on the measurement of tension. Distension of the abdominal cavity similarly has been used in measurement of laparotomy wounds and is subject to the same experimental variables.

Most studies of dermal or laparotomy wounds involve excision of the dermis or the abdominal wall containing the incision and measurement of breaking strength under uniaxial tension strips of measured width. Howes did this in his early work with the "Scott thread-testing machine." Subsequently, many investigators applied more gradual tension to wounds. This gradual distortion of the wound and skin leads to lower and more variable results because of slow disruption of the collagen matrix. Recent studies employ modern mechanical devices designed to measure tensile strength of materials by rapid disruption of the tissue and accurate tension measurements. Figure 3 demonstrates the increase in tensile strength of a dermal wound beginning about 7 days after injury.

Table 1. Models for assessment of wound healing

Model	Advantages	Disadvantages
Dermal wound	Single-layer closure produces consistent results	Effects of experimental variables in this model may not exactly duplicate changes in the more clinically important musculofascial layer
	Simple technique so large number of wounds can be tested	
Laparotomy (full thickness of abdominal wall or only musculofascial layer)	Clinically important wound because it is major source of strength after abdominal wound closures	Multiple-layer closure leads to increased variability in results Studies that use intrabdominal distension for measurement ignore law of Laplace
Enteric wound	Clinically important wound because of high morbidity of breakdown	Difficult to test accurately because of A. Thin walls and artifact of drying B. Error of bursting strength measurement because of law of Laplace C. Technically difficult anastomosis, and many studies have high frequency of leakage even in control groups

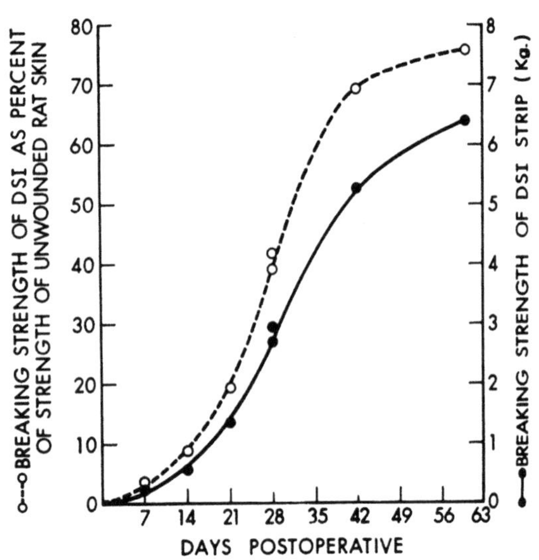

Fig. 3. Increase in breaking strength of a healing wound (rat skin), shown in absolute terms and as a percentage of the strength of comparable unwounded skin. This demonstrates the rapid rise in strength after the initial 7 days of healing. (Levenson et al. 1965)

Measurement of Sponge Collagen Deposition

Other methods of assessment of wound healing, in addition to the tensile strength of a wound, have been used. Boucek and Noble (1955) and Edwards et al. (1957) proposed the use of an implanted porous polyvinyl sponge as a means of isolating newly generated granulation tissue. These sponges demonstrated a sequence of histological events involving inflammatory cellular infiltration of the interstices and subsequent fibroblast migration, neovascularization, and collagen deposition, which followed a time course comparable to healing of an incised wound. The sponges provided a means of isolating granulation tissue that had been generated in a known period of time and that could be assayed free of surrounding "old" collagen. Studies have shown a good correlation between the amount of collagen deposited in the sponges and the tensile strength of normal wounds (Sandberg and Zederfeld 1963; Viljanto 1964).

Measurement of the Rate of Collagen Synthesis

Hydroxyproline is present almost exclusively in collagen, where proline is hydroxylated after its incorporation into a peptide chain (Juva 1968; Udenfriend 1966). Only trace amounts of hydroxyproline are present in acetylcholinesterase (Rosenberry and Richardson 1977), complement factor Clq (Porter 1977; Yonemasu et al. 1971), and elastin (Ross and Bornstein 1969). Thus, the tritiated hydroxyproline present in a wound following administration of tritiated proline is a direct measure of the newly synthesized collagen. Madden and Peacock (1967) first assessed the rate of collagen synthesis in an incised wound using this method. No increase in labeled hydroxyproline was demonstrated at 2 days after wounding, but by 4 days there was increased activity, which reached a maximum at 14 days and decreased gradually thereafter (Madden and Peacock 1967, 1968, 1971; Madden and Smith 1970) (Fig. 4). This clearly correlated with the histological onset of collagen deposition at 5–6 days, which had been previously described. Devereux et al. (1980c) used this technique to demonstrate the suppression of collagen synthesis as a result of doxorubicin (Adriamycin).

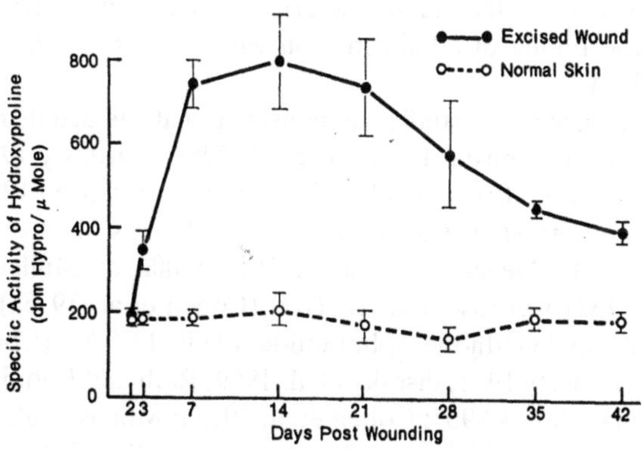

Fig. 4. Demonstration of the correlation between the interval after wound infliction and the rate of collagen synthesis measured by the production of hydroxyproline in an incised wound. Note the rapid rise in production between 4 and 7 days. (Madden and Peacock 1971)

Problems Specific to Chemotherapeutic Drug Studies

The experimental studies of chemotherapeutic agents on wound healing often appear to have contradictory results. These findings can often be explained by additional chemotherapy-related factors. Most information regarding the interaction between chemotherapy and wound healing is available from experimental studies in nonhuman subjects. The process of wound healing is similar in different species, so the variability in these studies arises not from species-specific differences in healing, but from a species-specific dose-response curve to the agent. Experimental studies must determine the systemic effects of the agent (death rate, weight loss, blood count, or oral intake) to define the relative dose used. Markedly different results occur with the same agent administered at different times relative to wounding. Wounds have been found to be most sensitive to impairment at the time of or immediately after injury. Progressively less impact occurs with increasing intervals between injury and administration (Calnan and Davis, Cohen et al. 1975b; Devereux et al. 1979b).

The route of administration, whether parenteral (IP, IV, or SC) or topical, determines the extent of both systemic and local effects of the agent and is an important factor in each study.

Most chemotherapeutic agents have systemic effects, including anorexia, weight loss, and anemia. To distinguish between direct impairment of healing by the agent or impairment secondary to one of the systemic abnormalities, appropriate controls must be included.

Thus, for adequate assessment of the results of studies of chemotherapeutic drugs and wound healing, we need to know species, wound site, dose, time of administration, route, method of assessing wound healing, systemic effects on the animal (food intake, weight loss, white cell count, hematocrit), and whether any local problems at the wound site (infection, perforation, or necrosis) occurred. The majority of studies fail to provide these data.

Antineoplastic Agents

Experimental studies have shown variable responses of wound healing to cytotoxic agents. The major factors that determine the extent of their effect are the agent and the dose used, the timing of administration with respect to wounding, and the nutritional state of the host.

Experimental studies demonstrate that the agents most detrimental to wound healing are nitrogen mustard (Farhat et al. 1958; Hardesty 1958; Hatiboglu et al. 1960), cyclophosphamide (Cohen et al. 1975b; Desprez and Kien 1960; Gupta et al. 1970; Wie et al. 1979), methotrexate (Calnan and Davies 1965; Cohen et al. 1975a), doxorubicin (Cohen et al. 1975b; Devereux et al. 1979a, 1980a, c; Mullen et al. 1981), and 1,3-bis(2-chloroethyl),1-nitrosourea (BCNU) (Cohen et al. 1975a). Variable or no effects occurred with triethylenethiophosphoramide (Thio-TEPA) (Conn et al. 1957; Farhat et al. 1959; Hardesty 1958; Pisesky et al. 1959; Rath and Enquist 1959), 5-fluorouracil (5-FU) (Calnan and Davies 1965; Cohen et al. 1975a; Morris et al. 1978; Paolucci et al. 1975; Staley et al. 1961), azathioprine (Arumugam et al. 1971), and vincristine (Cohen et al. 1975a). Mitomycin C (Paolucci et al. 1975; Wiznitzer et al. 1973), actinomycin D (Cohen et al. 1975a), bleomycin (Cohen et al. 1975a), and 6-mercaptopurine (Bole and Heath 1967) have not been adequately studied at this time to allow any firm statements regarding their effect (Table 2).

Table 2. Antineoplastic agents and wound healing

Agents clearly detrimental to wound healing	Nitrogen mustard Cyclophosphamide Methotrexate Doxorubicin (Adriamycin) 1,3- bis (2-chloroethyl)1-nitrosourea (BCNU)
Agents with variable or no effect on wound healing	Triethylene-thiophosphoramide (Thio-TEPA) 5-fluorouracil (5-FU) Azathioprine Vincristine
Agents inadequately studied for effect on wound healing to be assessed	Mitomycin C Actinomycin D Bleomycin 6-Mercaptopurine

The important role of dosage has been demonstrated with methotrexate (Calnan and Davies 1965) (Fig. 5), cyclophosphamide (Cohen et al. 1975b; Desprez and Kiehn 1960), and doxorubicin (Cohen et al. 1975b). Higher doses produce progressively greater impairment in healing. Administration of the agent within 4 days of the wounding has a greater effect on impairment with cyclophosphamide (Cohen et al. 1975b) and doxorubicin (Devereux et al. 1979a) (Figs. 6 and 7). Administration of these agents at a later time after wounding produces little effect, suggesting that they must be present during the early proliferative phase of healing to produce impairment. A similar situation may exist with other agents, but it has not been established.

A marked additive effect between nutritional deprivation and 5-FU has been demonstrated (Staley et al. 1961). Animals with a 20%–25% weight loss had a threefold decrease in wound strength when given 5-FU compared with animals given 5-FU while at their normal body weight. A similar effect may be present with other agents but has not been investigated.

Experimental studies with methotrexate have demonstrated a deleterious effect on the host's ability to tolerate contamination of a surgical wound (Ariyan et al. 1980a). This effect is greater with shorter time intervals between chemotherapy and wounding.

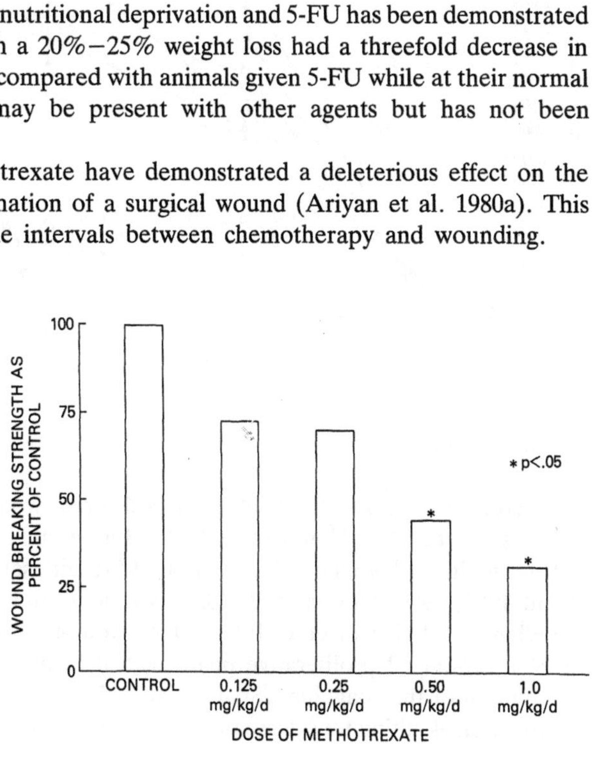

Fig. 5. Demonstration of the relationship between dose of methotrexate and decrease in wound breaking strength, shown as percentage of control. Methotrexate was administered IP for 5 days at these doses and strength measured at the 5th day. (Adapted from Calnan and Davies 1965)

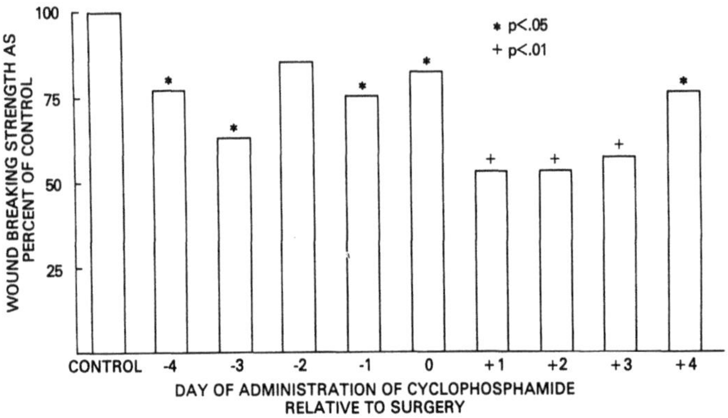

Fig. 6. Demonstration of the influence of time of administration of a single dose of cyclophosphamide (200 mg/kg) on the healing of dermal wounds in the mouse. Day-21 wound breaking strength is shown as a percentage of the control. Each group received a single injection on a different day from 4 days before injury (−4) to 4 days after injury (+4). (Adapted from Cohen et al. 1975b)

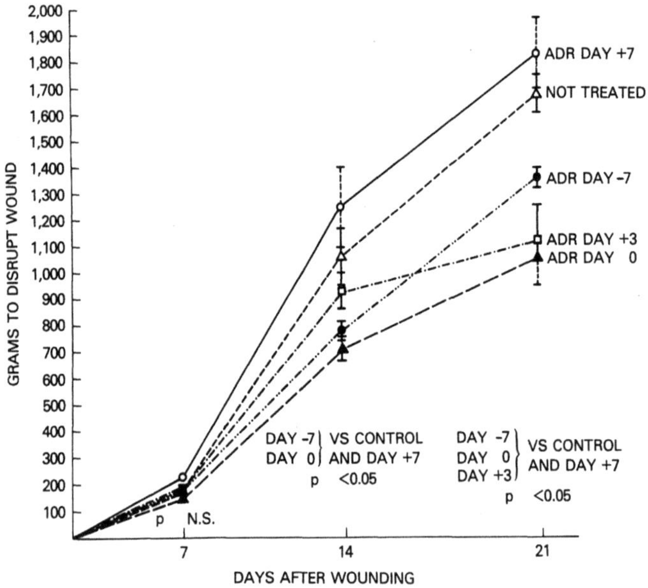

Fig. 7. Demonstration of the varying effect of doxorubicin *(ADR)* on wound tensile strength related to the time of administration. Administration of the drug 7 days before or a wounding was found to have created significant impairment when tested at 14 days, and both these modes and administration 3 days after wounding were found to have caused significant impairment when tested at 21 days. (Devereux et al. 1979a)

Corticosteroids

Corticosteroids impair the healing of both open wounds (Billingham and Russel 1956; Heite and Irro 1973; Howes et al. 1950; Hunt et al. 1969; Lenco et al. 1975; Spain et al. 1950) and incised wounds (Alrich et al. 1951; DiPasquale and Steinetz 1964; Ehrlich and Hunt 1968, 1969; Howes et al. 1950; Meadows and Prudden 1953; Pearce et al. 1960; Sandberg 1964; Taylor et al. 1952). Open wounds of animals treated with corticosteroids have a prolonged proliferative phase with delayed infiltration of cellular elements and dissolution of the coagulum (Spain et al. 1950). If corticosteroids are maintained wound contraction is ultimately decreased and epithelialization is delayed.

The importance of the dosage and timing of steroid administration must be stressed. If corticosteroids are begun 3 days or more after creation of an open wound, progression of cellular infiltration and the resulting fibroplasia are histologically unchanged (Spain et al. 1950). Similarly, corticosteroids begun 3–5 days after creation of an incised wound produce no effect on tensile strength (Sandberg 1964; Savlov et al. 1954), and some studies have shown that delayed administration (after 11 days) will actually improve tensile strength (tested over 21 days) (Vogel 1970). Histological studies of incised wounds in animals treated with steroids show "delayed infiltration" of "all cellular elements" (Alrich et al. 1951).

Dosage is also an important factor, in that small doses (5 mg/kg cortisone acetate per day in the rat) increase or have no effect on tensile strength, whereas higher doses significantly decrease tensile strength (Alrich et al. 1951; Arumugam et al. 1971; DiPasquale and Steinetz 1964; Findlay and Howes 1952; Meadows and Prudden 1953; Vogel 1970). The nutritional state also determines the sensitivity of the host. A dose of corticosteroids (cortisone 5 mg/kg per day SC) had no effect on the tensile strength of incised wounds in rabbits fed a regular diet or with limited feeding and a 3%–19% weight loss, but produced a marked inhibitory effect on tensile strength in rabbits with a 25%–35% weight loss (Findlay and Howes 1952). Again, a significant weight loss causes increased sensitivity in the host.

The impairment by steroids of healing of an incised wound is most obvious when tested at 7–14 days. By 3–4 weeks after injury the tensile strength approaches that of controls, indicating that the impaired healing results from a prolongation of the cellular phase (Vogel 1970). In the clinical setting administration of steroids in the perioperative period for "steroid coverage" should not be undertaken lightly. If adequate time is available to measure cortisol levels before and after ACTH stimulation it should be done, to avoid excessive use of these agents. If there are clear-cut indications for their use in the emergency setting, the wound should be considered at increased risk for complications.

Radiotherapy

Radiotherapy impairs the healing of dermal and visceral wounds in experimental studies (Dobbs 1939; Grillo 1963; Grillo and Potsaid 1961; Hunt and Pai 1972; Lawrence et al. 1953; Murphy et al. 1980; Stajie and Milovanovic 1970; Zelman et al. 1969). This is a direct effect on exposed tissues, and healing at distal sites is normal unless significant weight loss results from the radiation. The effect is dose related, with small doses having no effect (Nathanson 1934; Stajie and Milovanovic 1970; Zelman et al. 1969). The pathophysiology of this impairment is probably a combination of direct injury to the fibroblasts and endothelial tissues (Rudolph et al. 1981). Studies have demonstrated both a lower collagen content of radiated skin and a decreased rate of collagen production by radiated wounds (Archer et al. 1970; Kitagawa et al. 1961). In the early, proliferative phase of healing fibroblast division is an integral component of scar formation. Radiation injury to chromatin would blunt this response. Histological studies of wounds exposed to a single dose of radiation (10 Gy, 100 kV) at 24 or 48 hours after injury demonstrate a "sluggish" cellular response to the injury (Pohle and Ritchie 1933). This effect is less marked if radiation is given prior to injury (Pohle et al. 1931; Ritchie 1933).

Progressive fibrosis of vessels occurs as a delayed result following radiation. Decreased blood flow to the tissue and a lower level of oxygen saturation would result. Oxygen gradients have been demonstrated across healing wounds and are felt to be a major determinant in healing (Niinikoski et al. 1972; Remensnyder and Majno 1968). Studies of animals maintained in hypoxic environments have demonstrated decreased DNA in the healing tissues, slower accumulation of wound collagen, and more slowly increasing wound breaking strength (Grillo and Potsaid 1961; Hunt and Pai 1972; Stephens and Hunt 1971). Impaired perfusion of surrounding tissues resulting from endothelial fibrosis would have a similar effect.

Incised wounds in radiated tissues, when experimentally contaminated, become infected more frequently than do wounds in normal tissues (Ariyan et al. 1980b). This susceptibility to infections has been observed clinically. Infection would predispose the wound to higher rates of dehiscence and failure and decreased wound breaking strength, as has been demonstrated experimentally (Fu 1979; Phillips and Fu 1976).

Systemic chemotherapy, primarily doxorubicin and actinomycin D can produce ulcerations in areas previously treated with radiation. This radiation recall phenomenon suggests that irradiated fibroblasts have permanently impaired synthetic or proliferative function. When tissues are exposed to these agents and radiotherapy even sequentially, they are unable to maintain their integrity. Studies in vitro of mammalian cells exposed to doxorubicin and radiation have demonstrated that they produce independent classes of damage to the cells (Belli and Piro 1977). Doxorubicin does not bring about radiosensitivity of the cells or their repair of sublethal radiation damage. This is not found with any other chemotherapeutic agents. Combined radiation and doxorubicin have an additive impairment on wound healing in the experimental animal. This results in lower production of wound collagen and decreased wound breaking strength (Fig. 8) (Devereux et al. 1980a).

Mechanisms of Action

The etiology of wound healing impairment by chemotherapeutic agents has not been established. Several mechanisms have been explored and will be discussed briefly. It is hoped that when the mechanism of injury is understood its occurrence can be prevented.

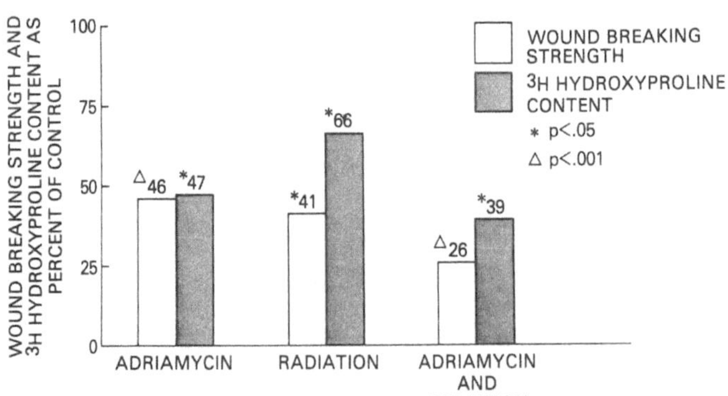

Fig. 8. Impairment of wound breaking strength and ^{3}H-hydroxyproline production in a 21-day wound, shown as a percentage of the control values for doxorubicin (*Adriamycin*) 6 mg/kg, radiation (single dose 20 Gy), and both agents combined. An additive effect of their combined application was demonstrated. (Adapted from Devereux et al. 1980a)

Effect of Leukopenia on Wound Healing

The leukopenia induced by chemotherapy has been a prominent suspect in the impairment of wound healing. This suspicion has not been supported by experimental work. Contaminated wounds are more likely to become infected after administration of chemotherapeutic agents (Ariyan et al. 1980a; Kraft et al. 1979), but minimal problems were encountered with clean wounds in any of the experimental studies.

Several authors have used antineutrophil serum (ANS) to study the effect of neutropenia on wound healing. Simpson and Ross (1972) compared such wounds histologically with control wounds and found there were no neutrophils in the wound space though a normal volume of mononuclear leukocytes was present in the coagulum. Despite the absence of neutrophils, there was a normal progression of wound debridement and repair at 10 days. This was supported by Stein and Levenson (1966), who showed normal wound strength and polyvinyl sponge collagen content at 5 days in similarly treated animals. In addition, Wiener (1976, 1977), studying the granulation tissue induced around a polyvinyl sponge, showed no decrease in thymidine uptake by activated fibroblasts or decrease in prolyl hydroxylase in animals that were neutropenic as a result of ANS (Wiener et al. 1976, 1977).

Lymphocytopenia failed to affect wound healing in lymphopenic rats. A normal inflammatory response at 24 and 48 hours was demonstrated by histological study, and normal wound strength and sponge collagen content were found at 7 and 14 days. Rats made leukopenic by the administration of cyclophosphamide failed to demonstrate any suppression of fibroblast DNA synthesis or prolyl hydroxylase activation of granulation tissue induced by polyvinyl sponges and tested in vitro (Wiener et al. 1976, 1977). Thus, neutropenia, lymphopenia, or leukopenia alone fails to suppress wound healing as assessed by histological and biochemical techniques.

Effect of Macrophages on Wound Healing

The macrophage plays a critical role in wound healing (Diegelmann et al. 1981). Leibovich and Ross (1975) performed a morphological study in guinea pigs of the effect of locally injected antimacrophage serum (AMS) around the wound or the administration of systemic hydrocortisone. The local injections of AMS had no effect on circulating monocytes or on the number or phagocytic action of the wound macrophages. Systemic hydrocortisone induced prolonged monocytopenia, and the macrophage level in the wounds was approximately one-third that of controls. Mild inhibition of wound debridement was observed, but collagen synthesis was similar to that of control wounds. Combined AMS and hydrocortisone resulted in almost complete absence of wound macrophages and clearance of debris was decreased, fibroblasts appeared later, and 7- to 10-day wounds appeared immature compared with controls in terms of collagen synthesis. Studies by Hunt's group have shown in two systems, a rabbit ear chamber and a corneal injection model, that the presence of wound macrophages or stimulated peritoneal macrophages enhances neovascularization in both systems (Clark et al. 1976; Thakral et al. 1979). Polverini et al. (1977) studied the effects of monocytes on neovascularization in the avascular guinea pig cornea. "Activated" macrophages (peritoneal macrophages from animals treated with paraffin oil or thioglycollate IP) resulted in a high frequency of neovascularization, whereas "unactivated" macrophages infrequently generated a response. Media from cultures of "activated" macrophages had an intermediate response.

Implantation of polymorphonuclear cells or activated lymphocytes produced no neovascularization in this system.
Injection into the dermis and subcutaneous tissues of peritoneal macrophages immediately before wounding leads to increased wound breaking strength at 8 days (Casey et al. 1976). Thus, the macrophage appears to play an important role in the clearance of wound debris and neovascularization of the wound space. Susceptibility of the macrophages to specific chemotherapeutic drugs has not been demonstrated, but may occur, particularly with agents that are active when giving during or before the cellular phase (days 1–4). This may be one major site of suppression of healing induced by corticosteroids.

Effects of Nutritional Depletion on Wound Healing

Up to two-thirds of patients develop cancer cachexia during the course of their illness. In many cases this occurs late in their disease, yet a surgical procedure is often required after the onset of significant weight loss. Caloric and protein depletion of experimental animals is an established inhibitor of dermal, musculofascial, and visceral healing, but only after a loss of 15%–20% of the body weight (Daly et al. 1972).
A direct impairment of wound healing by the tumor has been proposed. This decrease in wound healing, however, may be entirely due to the weight loss resulting from the tumor. In experimental studies tumor-bearing animals have a decrease in wound breaking strength only after a 15%–20% decrease in carcass weight (Devereux et al. 1979b). Decreases in wound breaking strength are proportional to the carcass weight loss. Excision of the tumor early in its growth, before a significant carcass weight loss has occurred, will preserve normal healing (Devereux et al. 1980b).

Effect of Anemia on Wound Healing

Patients with malignancies are frequently anemic. Experimental studies of anemia induced by phlebotomy or iron-deficient diets have shown a suppression of wound healing only in the presence of volume deficit or significant malnutrition associated with the iron-deficient diet (Bains et al. 1966; Jacobson and Prohaska 1965). Anemia resulting from phlebotomy with volume replacement or repeated drawings of smaller volumes results in normal healing (Heughan et al. 1974; Hugo et al. 1969; Macon and Pones 1971; Sandberg and Zederfeldt 1959). Anemia should not be expected to be a factor in suppressed wound healing.

Conclusion

This summary of available reports indicates that patients with malignant disease who have a significant weight loss (15%–20%), have recently received cytotoxic agents, are receiving glucocorticoids, or have received radiotherapy in the area of their wound are at increased risk for complications of wound healing. Steps currently available to avoid these complications are limited. It is suggested that temporary improvement of the nutritional state of the patient may lower the frequency of complications, but this needs support from further studies.

Avoidance of operations immediately after chemotherapy is important. Current adjuvant chemotherapy studies are now designed with treatment delayed until 7–10 days after surgery, based on the results of experimental studies.

The possibility of stimulating wound healing has intrigued many surgeons. The normal wound has often been considered a "privileged site" where healing can occur even if the entire organism is in a catabolic state (Moore and Brennan 1975). Despite much research in the area, few factors have been found that will accelerate the rate of normal healing. Exposure to hyperbaric oxygen will accelerate healing (Hunt and Pai 1972; Stephens and Hunt), but exogenous vitamin C or vitamin A (Ehrlich and Hunt 1968) in a normal host does not demonstrate the salutary effect either has in scorbutic (Bartlett et al. 1942a, b), diabetic (Seifter et al. 1981), or corticosteroid-treated subjects (Ehrlich and Hunt 1968; Ehrlich et al. 1973; Salmela and Ahonen 1981). Reversal of impairment caused by methotrexate was achieved with leucovorin (Fig. 9), but as in other studies, leucovorin in the normal host provided no benefit (Calnan and Davies 1965). Such specific "rescue" agents are needed for other chemotherapeutic drugs. Vitamin E and *N*-acetylcysteine reversal of doxorubin-induced impairment was attempted but failed (Fig. 10). Trials of anabolic steroids for reversal of inhibition caused by corticosteroids (Ehrlich and Hunt 1969; Pearce et al. 1960), cyclophosphamide (Desprez and Kiehn 1960; Gupta et al. 1970), and thio-TEPA (Pisesky et al. 1959) have provided variable results, and no clear-cut

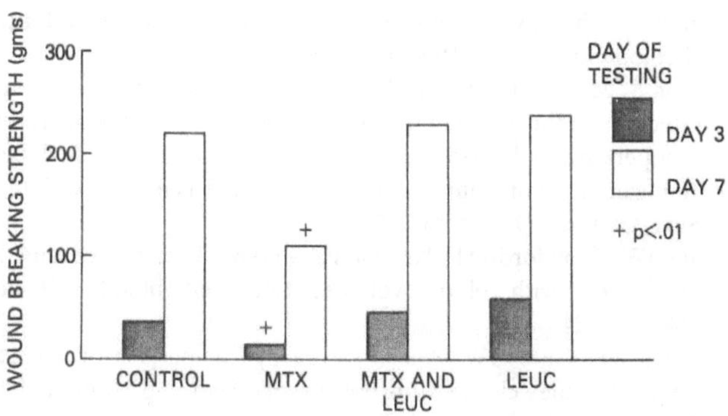

Fig. 9. The ability of leucovorin (*LEUC*) to reverse the impairment by methotrexate (*MTX*) of wound breaking strength is shown for wounds tested at both 3 and 7 days after wounding. (Adapted from Calnan and Davies 1965)

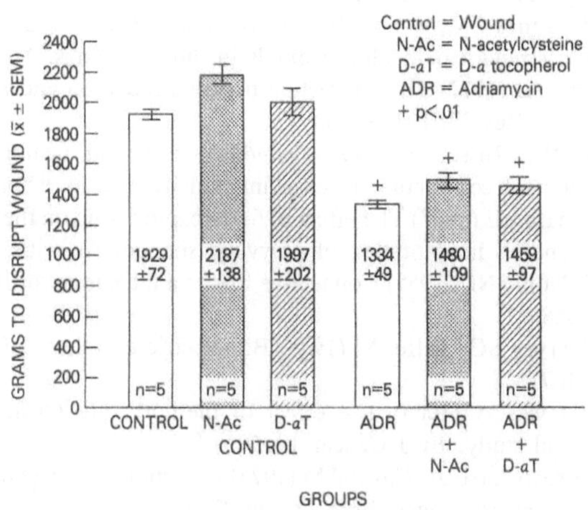

Fig. 10. Reversal of doxorubicin (*ADR*) impairment of wound tensile strength was not achieved by administration of *N*-acetylcysteine (*N-Ac*) or *D-α*-tocopheral (*D-αT*), as shown for 21-day wounds (Devereux et al., unpublished data)

benefit can be attributed to them at this time. A preliminary report suggests that vitamin A administration can at least partially reverse the impairment produced by cyclophosphamide (Stratford et al. 1980). This will merit further investigation with additional cytotoxic agents.

The data provided above give some insight into the pathophysiology of abnormal wound healing in the cancer patients. Obvious gaps exist in our knowledge regarding the effects of specific agents and the mechanism of their effect. More importantly, once a wound at particular risk for abnormal healing is identified, we have little at our disposal to stimulate healing. More work must be undertaken in this area.

References

Ahonen J (1968) Nucleic acids in experimental granuloma. Acta Physiol Scand [Suppl] 315: 1–73

Alrich EM, Carter JP, Lehman EP (1951) The effect of ACTH and cortisone on wound healing. Ann Surg 133: 783–789

Archer RR, Greenwell EJ, Ware T, Weeks PM (1970) Irradiation effect on wound healing in rats. Radiat Res 41: 104–112

Ariyan S, Kraft RL, Goldberg NH (1980a) An experimental model to determine the effects of adjuvant therapy on the incidence of postoperative wound infection: II. Evaluating preoperative chemotherapy. Plast Reconstr Surg 65: 338–345

Ariyan S, Marfuggi RA, Harder G, Goodie MM (1980b) An experimental model to determine the effects of adjuvant therapy on the incidence of postoperative wound infection: I. Evaluating preoperative radiation therapy. Plast Reconstr Surg 65: 328–337

Arumugam S, Nimmannit S, Enquist IF (1971) The effect of immunosuppression on wound healing. Surg Gynecol Obstet 133: 72–74

Bains JW, Crawford DT, Ketcham AS (1966) Effect of chronic anemia on wound tensile strength: correlation with blood volume, total red blood cell volume and proteins. Ann Surg 164: 243–246

Barham RE, Butz GW, Ansell JS (1978) Comparison of wound strength in normal, radiated and infected tissues closed with polyglycolic acid and chromic catgut sutures. Surg Gynecol Obstet 146: 901–907

Bartlett MK, Jones CM, Ryan AE (1942a) Vitamin C and wound healing I. Experimental wounds in guinea pigs. N Engl J Med 226: 469–473

Bartlett MK, Jones CM, Ryan AE (1942b) Vitamin C and wound healing II. Ascorbic acid content and tensile strength of healing wounds in human beings. N Engl J Med 226: 474–481

Belli JA, Piro AJ (1977) The interaction between radiation and Adriamycin damage in mammalian cells. Cancer Res 37: 1624–1630

Billingham RE, Russell PS (1956) Studies on wound healing, with special reference to the phenomenon of contracture in experimental wounds in rabbits' skin. Ann Surg 144: 961–981

Bole GG, Heath LE (1967) The effect of 6-mercaptopurine on the inflammatory response stimulated by subcutaneous implantation of polyvinyl sponge. Arthritis Rheum 10: 377–387

Boucek RJ, Noble NL (1955) Connective tissue: a technique for its isolation and study. Arch Pathol 59: 553–558

Burr HS, Harvey SC, Taffel M (1938) Bio-electric correlates of wound healing. Yale J Biol Med 11: 103–107

Calnan J, Davies A (1965) The effect of methotrexate (Amethopterin) on wound healing: an experimental study. Br J Cancer 19: 505–512

Casey WJ, Peacock EE Jr, Chvapil M (1976) Induction of collagen synthesis in rats by transplantation of allogenic macrophages. Surg Forum 27: 53–55

Clark RA, Stone RD, Leung DYK, Silver I, Hohn DC, Hunt TK (1976) Role of macrophages in wound healing. Surg Forum 27: 16–18

Cohen SC, Gabelnick HL, Johnson RK, Goldin A (1975a) Effects of antineoplastic agents on wound healing in mice. Surgery 78: 238–244

Cohen SC, Gabelnick HL, Johnson RK, Goldin A (1975b) Effects of cyclophosphamide and Adriamycin on the healing of surgical wounds in mice. Cancer 36: 1277–1281

Conn JH, Leb SM, Hardy JD (1957) Effect of nitrogen mustard and thio-TEPA on wound healing. Surg Forum 8: 80–83

Cuthbertson DP (1954) Interrelationship of metabolic changes consequent to injury. Br Med Bull 10: 33–37

Daly JM, Vars HM, Dudrick SJ (1972) Effects of protein depletion on strength of colonic anastomoses. Surg Gynecol Obstet 134: 15–21

Desprez JD, Kiehn CL (1960) The effects of cytoxan (cyclophosphamide) on wound healing. Plast Reconstr Surg 26: 301–308

Devereux DF, Thibault L, Boretos J, Brennan MF (1979a) The quantitative and qualitative impairment of wound healing by Adriamycin. Cancer 43: 932–938

Devereux DF, Thistlethwaite PA, Thibault LE, Brennan MF (1979b) Effects of tumor bearing and protein depletion on wound breaking strength in the rat. J Surg Res 27: 233–238

Devereux DF, Kent H, Brennan MF (1980a) Time dependent effects of Adriamycin and X-ray therapy on wound healing in the rat. Cancer 45: 2805–2810

Devereux DF, Thibault L, Brennan MF (1980b) Effects of tumor removal on wound breaking strength in rats. Surg Forum 31: 234–236

Devereux DF, Triche TJ, Webber BL, Thibault LE, Brennan MF (1980c) A study of Adriamycin-reduced wound breaking strength in rats: an evaluation by light and electron microscopy, induction of collagen maturation, and hydroxyproline content. Cancer 45: 2811–2815

Diegelmann RF, Cohen IK, Kaplan AM (1981) The role of macrophages in wound repair: a review. Plast Reconstr Surg 68: 107–113

DiPasquale G, Steinetz BG (1964) Relationship of food intake to the effect of cortisone acetate on skin wound healing. Proc Soc Exp Biol Med 117: 118–121

Dobbs WGH (1939) A statistical study of the effect of roentgen rays on wound healing. AJR 41: 625–632

Dunphy JE, Jackson DS (1962) Practical applications of experimental studies in the care of the primarily closed wound. Am J Surg 104: 273–282

Dunphy JE, Udupa KN (1955) Chemical and histochemical sequences in the normal healing of wounds. N Engl J Med 253: 847–851

Edwards LC, Pernokas LN, Dunphy JE (1957) The use of a plastic sponge to sample regenerating tissue in healing wounds. Surg Gynecol Obstet 105: 303–309

Ehrlich HP, Hunt TK (1968) Effects of cortisone and vitamin A on wound healing. Ann Surg 169: 324–328

Ehrlich HP, Hunt TK (1969) The effects of cortisone and anabolic steroids on the tensile strength of healing wounds. Ann Surg 170: 203–206

Ehrlich HP, Tarver H, Hunt TK (1963) Effects of vitamin A and glucocorticoids upon inflammation and collagen synthesis. Ann Surg 177: 222–227

Farhat SM, Amer NS, Weeks DS, Musselman MM (1958) Effect of mechlorethamine hydrochloride (nitrogen mustard) on healing of abdominal wounds. Arch Surg 76: 749–753

Farhat SM, Miller DM, Musselman MM (1959) Effect of triethylenethiophosphoramide (Thio-TEPA) upon healing of abdominal wounds. Arch Surg 78: 729–731

Findlay CW Jr, Howes EL (1952) The combined effect of cortisone and partial protein depletion on wound healing. N Engl J Med 246: 597–604

Fu KK (1979) Normal tissue effects of combined radiotherapy and chemotherapy for head and neck cancer. Front Radiat Ther Oncol 13: 113–132

Grillo HC (1963) Origin of fibroblasts in wound healing: an autoradiographic study of inhibition of cellular proliferation by local X-irradiation. Ann Surg 157: 453–467

Grillo HC, Potsaid MS (1961) Studies in wound healing: IV. retardation of contraction by local X-irradiation, and observations relating to the origin of fibroblasts in repair. Ann Surg 154: 741–750
Gupta RC, Singh LM, Udupa KN (1970) Effect of cyclophosphamide (Endoxan) on the process of wound healing. Indian J Surg 32: 127–132
Hardesty WH (1958) The effect of cytotoxic drugs on wound healing in rats. Cancer Res 18: 581–584
Hatiboglu I, Moore GE, Wilkens HJ, Hoffmeister F (1960) Effects of chemotherapeutic agents on wounds contaminated with tumor cells: an experimental study. Ann Surg 152: 559–567
Heite VHJ, Irro H (1973) Ablauf der wundheilung unter anwendung anaboler und kataboler steroide am kaninchenohr-modell nach Heite. Arzneimittelforsch 23: 1341–1346
Heughan C, Grislis G, Hunt TK (1974) The effect of anemia on wound healing. Ann Surg 179: 163–167
Howes EL, Sooy JW, Harvey SC (1929) The healing of wounds as determined by their tensile strength. JAMA 92: 42–45
Howes EL, Ploth CM, Blunt JW, Ragan C (1950) Retardation of wound healing by cortisone. Surgery 28: 177–181
Hugo NE, Thompson LW, Zook EG, Bennett JE (1969) Effect of chronic anemia on the tensile strength of healing wounds. Surgery 66: 741–745
Hunt TK, Pai MP (1972) The effect of varying ambient oxygen tensions on wound metabolism and collagen synthesis. Surg Gynecol Obstet 135: 561–567
Hunt TK, Ehrlich HP, Garcia JA, Dunphy JE (1969) Effect of vitamin A on reversing the inhibitory effect of cortisone on healing of open wounds in animals and man. Ann Surg 170: 633–641
Jacobson MJ, Prohaska JV (1965) The healing of wounds in iron deficiency. Surgery 57: 254–258
Juva K (1968) Hydroxylation of proline in the biosynthesis of collagen. Acta Physiol Scand [Suppl] 308: 1–73
Kitagawa T, Glicksman AS, Tyree EB, Nickson JJ (1961) Radiation effects on skin and subcutaneous tissue. A quantitative study of collagen content: modification with L-triiodothyronine. Radiat Res 15: 761–766
Kraft RL, Goldberg NH, Ariyan S (1979) Effect of preoperative high-dose methotrexate and leucovorin rescue on incidence of wound infection in rats. Surg Forum 30: 537–539
Lawrence W Jr, Nickson JJ, Washaw LM (1953) Roentgen rays and wound healing. An experimental study. Surgery 33: 376–384
Leibovich SJ, Ross R (1975) The role of the macrophage in wound repair: a study with hydrocortisone and antimacrophage serum. Am J Pathol 78: 71–99
Lenco W, McKnight M, MacDonald AS (1975) Effects of cortisone acetate, methylprednisolone and medroxyprogesterone on wound contracture and epithelization in rabbits. Ann Surg 181: 67–73
Levenson SM, Crowley LV, Geever EF, Rosen H, Berard CW (1964) Some studies of wound healing: experimental methods, effect of ascorbic acid and effect of deuterium oxide. J Trauma 4: 543–566
Levenson SM, Geever EF, Crowley LV, Oates JF III, Berard CW, Rosen H (1965) The healing of rat skin wounds. Ann Surg 161: 293–308
Macon WL, Pories WJ (1971) The effect of iron deficiency anemia on wound healing. Surgery 69: 792–796
Madden JW, Peacock EE Jr (1967) Measurement of the rate of collagen synthesis in sutured rat wounds. Surg Forum 18: 56–57
Madden JW, Peacock EE Jr (1968) Studies on the biology of collagen during wound healing. I. Rate of collagen synthesis and deposition in cutaneous wounds of the rat. Surgery 64: 288–294
Madden JW, Peacock EE Jr (1971) Studies on the biology of collagen during wound healing: III. Dynamic metabolism of scar collagen and remodeling of dermal wounds. Ann Surg 174: 511–520

Madden JW, Smith HC (1970) The rate of collagen synthesis and deposition in dehisced and resutured wounds. Surg Gynecol Obstet 130: 487–493

Meadows EC, Prudden JF (1953) A study of the influence of adrenal steroids on the strength of healing wounds. Surgery 33: 841–848

Moore FD, Brennan MF (1975) Surgical injury: body composition, protein metabolism, and neuroendocrinology. In: Ballinger WF, Collins JA, Drucker WR, Dudrick SJ, Zeppa R (eds) Manual of surgical nutrition. Saunders, Philadelphia, pp 172–173

Morris T, Lincoln F, Lee A (1978) The effect of 5-fluorouracil on abdominal wound healing in rats. Aust NZ J Surg 48: 219–221

Mullen BM, Mattox DE, Von Hoff DD, Hearne EM (1981) The effect of preoperative adriamycin and dihydroxyanthracenedione on wound healing. Laryngoscope 91: 1436–1443

Murphy K, Frith C, Lang N, Westbrook KC (1980) Effect of radiotherapy on healing of colonic anastomoses. Surg Forum 31: 222–223

Nathanson IT (1934) The effect of the gamma-ray of radium on wound healing. Surg Gynecol Obstet 59: 62–69

Niinikoski J (1969) Effect of oxygen supply on wound healing and formation of experimental granulation tissue. Acta Physiol Scand [Suppl] 334: 7

Niinikoski J, Hunt TK, Dunphy JE (1972) Oxygen supply in healing tissue. Am J Surg 123: 247–252

Paolucci R, Zanoni F, Azzarelli A (1975) L'azione della chemioterapia sui processi di cicatrizzazione. Tumori 61: 441–446

Pearce CW, Foot NC, Jordan GL Jr, Law SW, Wantz GE Jr (1960) The effect and interrelation of testosterone, cortisone, and protein nutrition on wound healing. Surg Gynecol Obstet 111: 274–284

Phillips TL, Fu KK (1976) Quantification of combined radiation therapy and chemotherapy effects on critical normal tissues. Cancer 37: 1186–1200

Pisesky W, Williams HTG, MacKenzie WC (1959) The effect of triethylene thiophosphoramide (ThioTEPA) and 17-ethyl-19-nortestosterone (Nilevar) on wound healing. Can J Surg 2: 291–294

Pohle EA, Ritchie G (1933) Studies of the effect of roentgen rays on the healing of wounds II. Histological changes in skin wounds in rats following postoperative irradiation. Radiology 20: 102–108

Pohle EA, Ritchie G, Wright CS (1931) Studies of the effect of roentgen rays on the healing of wounds I. The behavior of skin wounds in rats under pre- or post-operative irradiation. Radiology 16: 445–460

Polverini PJ, Cotran RS, Gimbrone MA Jr, Unanue ER (1977) Activated macrophages induce vascular proliferation. Nature 269: 804–806

Porter RR (1977) Structure and activation of early components of complement. Fed Proc 36: 2191–2196

Rath H, Enquist IF (1959) The effect of Thio-TEPA on wound healing. Arch Surg 79: 812–814

Remensnyder JP, Majno G (1968) Oxygen gradients in healing wounds. Am J Pathol 52: 301–323

Ritchie G (1933) Effect of roentgen irradiation on the healing of wounds. Arch Pathol 16: 839–851

Rosenberrry TL, Richardson JM (1977) Structure of 18S and 14S acetylcholinesterase. Identification of collagen-like subunits that are linked by disulfide bonds to catalytic subunits. Biochemistry 16: 3550–3558

Ross R, Benditt EP (1962) Wound healing and collagen formation II. Fine structure in experimental scurvy. J Cell Biol 12: 533–551

Ross R, Bornstein P (1969) The elastic fiber I. The separation and partial characterization of its macromolecular components. J Cell Biol 40: 366–381

Rudolph R, Utley J, Woodward M, Hurn I (1981) The ultrastructure of chronic radiation damage in rat skin. Surg Gynecol Obstet 152: 171–178

Salmela K, Ahonen J (1981) The effect of methylprednisolone and vitamin A on wound healing. Acta Chir Scand 147: 307–312
Sandberg N (1964) Time relationship between administration of cortisone and wound healing in rats. Acta Chir Scand 127: 446–455
Sandberg N, Zederfeldt B (1959) Influence of acute hemorrhage on wound healing in the rabbit. Acta Chir Scand 118: 367–371
Sandberg N, Zederfeldt B (1963) The tensile strength of healing wounds and collagen formation in rats and rabbits. Acta Chir Scand 126: 187–196
Savlov ED, Dunphy JE, Anderson MA (1954) The healing of the disrupted and resutured wound. Surgery 36: 362–370
Seifter E, Rettura G, Padawer J, Stratford F, Kambosos D, Levenon SM (1981) Impaired wound healing in streptozotocin diabetes. Prevention by supplemental vitamin A. Ann Surg 194: 42–50
Simpson DM, Ross R (1972) The neutrophilic leukocyte in wound repair. A study with antineutrophil serum. J Clin Invest 51: 2009–2023
Spain DM, Molomut N, Haber A (1950) Biological studies on cortison in mice. Science 112: 335–337
Stajie J, Milovanovic A (1970) Radiation and wound healing: evolution of tensile strength in excised skin-wound of irradiated rats. Strahlentherapie 139: 87–90
Staley CJ, Trippel OH, Preston FW (1961) Influence of 5-fluorouracil on wound healing. Surgery 49: 450–453
Stein JM, Levenson SM (1966) Effect of the inflammatory reaction on subsequent wound healing. Surg Forum 17: 484–485
Stephens FO, Hunt TK (1971) Effect of changes in inspired oxygen and carbon dioxide tensions on wound tensile strength: an experimental study. Ann Surg 173: 515–519
Stratford F, Seifter E, Rettura G, Babyatsky M, Levenson SM (1980) Impaired wound healing due to cyclophosphamide alleviated by supplemental vitamin A. Surg Forum 31: 224–225
Taylor FW, Dittmer TL, Porter DO (1952) Wound healing and the steroids. Surgery 31: 683–690
Thakral KK, Goodson WH III, Hunt TK (1979) Stimulation of wound blood vessel growth by wound macrophages. J Surg Res 26: 430–436
Udenfriend S (1966) Formation of hydroxyproline in collagen. Science 152: 1335–1340
Viljanto J (1964) Biochemical basis of tensile strength in wound healing. Acta Chir Scand [Suppl] 333: 1–91
Vogel HG (1970) Tensile strength of skin wounds in rats after treatment with corticosteroids. Acta Endocrinol 64: 295–303
Wie H, Bruaset I, Eckersberg T (1979) Effects of cyclophosphamide an open granulating skin wounds in rats. Acta Pathol Microbiol Scand [A] 87: 185–192
Wiener SL, Urivetsky M, Isenberg HD, Havier R, Wiener R, Belenko M, Heydu E, Meilman E (1976) Fibroblast DNA synthesis activation in sponge induced granulation tissue: the effect of antineutrophil serum and cyclophosphamide. Connect Tissue Res 4: 223–235
Wiener SL, Urivetsky M, Isenberg HD, Belenko M, Talansky A, Havier R, Meilman E (1977) Activation of prolyl hydroxylase in sponge induced granulation tissue: the effect of antineutrophil serum and inhibitor drugs. Connect Tissue Res 5: 97–108
Wiznitzer T, Orda R, Bawnik JB, Rippin A, Griffel B, Herzberg M (1973) Mitomycin and the healing of intestinal anastomosis: an experimental study in the rat. Arch Surg 106: 314–316
Yonemasu K, Stroud RM, Niedermeier W, Butler WT (1971) Chemical studies on Clq; A modulator of immunoglobulin biology. Biochem Biophys Res Commun 43: 1388–1394
Zelman D, Song IC, Porteous DD, Bromberg BE (1969) The effect of total body irradiation on wound healing and the hematopoietic system in mice. Bull NY Acad Med 45: 293–300

Influence of Perioperative cis-Platinum on Breaking Strength of Bowel Anastomoses in Rats

U. Engelmann, W. Sonntag, and G. H. Jacobi

Urologische Klinik und Poliklinik, Johannes-Gutenberg-Universität Mainz,
Langenbeckstrasse 1, 6500 Mainz, Germany

Introduction

Adjuvant and perioperative chemotherapy is increasingly being used in the treatment of malignant disease. Therefore, the influence of cytostatic drugs is of interest and is being investigated experimentally. The influence of various drugs is well known and has been described elsewhere (Shamberger et al. 1981). Recently, *cis*-platinum, an inorganic complex that inhibits DNA synthesis by cross-linking DNA strands, has been introduced. In urology it has shown a surprisingly good effect on testicular tumors and has been used in bladder cancer for palliative treatment, being one of the most potent drugs for this purpose (Yagoda 1979). It is now being combined with cystectomy for curative therapy (Merrin 1981). Because ileal or colon conduits are frequently combined with cystectomy, the potential effect of *cis*-platinum on bowel anastomosis is of interest. Our clinical findings with perioperative treatment with *cis*-platinum have suggested a negative influence of the drug on bowel anastomosis in a limited number of patients.

Materials and Methods

For the investigations of wound breaking strength (WBS) we used 104 male Sprague-Dawley rats, a further 70 being used for light microscopy and microangiography. They received *cis*-platinum in a dose of 5 mg/kg body weight IV on day −1 or day −5 preoperatively. In each animal, a small- and a large-bowel anastomosis was performed. In these investigations, WBS was measured with a material tester from the Institute of Physiology, and we now use an Instron material tester. Measurements were taken on days +4, +7, +14, and +28 postoperatively. Histological sections were stained with H & E, van Gieson, and PAS and examined by light microscopy. Microangiograms were performed with micropaque and a Diagnost M (Philips).

Operative Technique

The bowel was cut, not resected, and the mesentery was not damaged. The anastomoses were constructed with single-layer everted 6/0 sutures. For measurements, 4-mm-wide strips were used. Until investigation they were kept moist with saline solution. The

Recent Results in Cancer Research. Vol. 98

unilateral cross-speed of the material tester was 4 mm/min; the graph speed was 2 cm/min.

Results

The results in small-bowel anastomoses are shown in Fig. 1. The WBS of intact bowel lies between 100 and 125 lb. On day +4 the WBS in the control group was very low, while the WBS of the treatment group was not measurable.

On day +7 the control group reached a breaking strength of 34 lb and the treatment groups reached 26 lb and 16 lb. The difference was most pronounced on day +14 postoperatively, with a breaking strength of 71 lb in the control group and about 25–29 lb in the treatment groups. After 4 weeks all groups had reached near-normal values.

The results in the large-bowel anastomoses are shown in Fig. 2.

On day +4 the values in the control group were low and the values of the treatment groups not measurable. On day +7 the treatment groups that received *cis*-platinum on day −1 had almost the same results as the nontreatment groups, whereas the animals which had

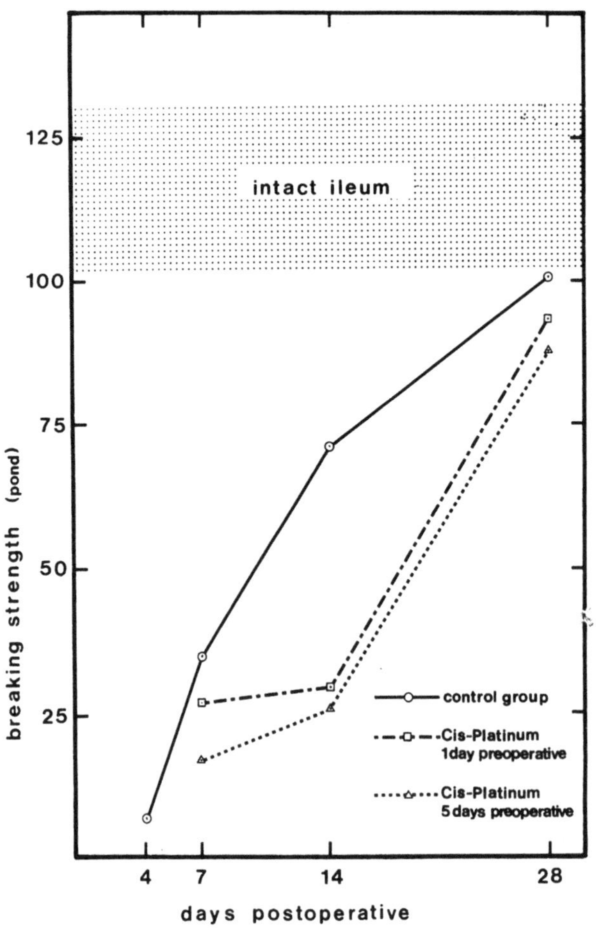

Fig. 1. WBS in the small-bowel anastomoses

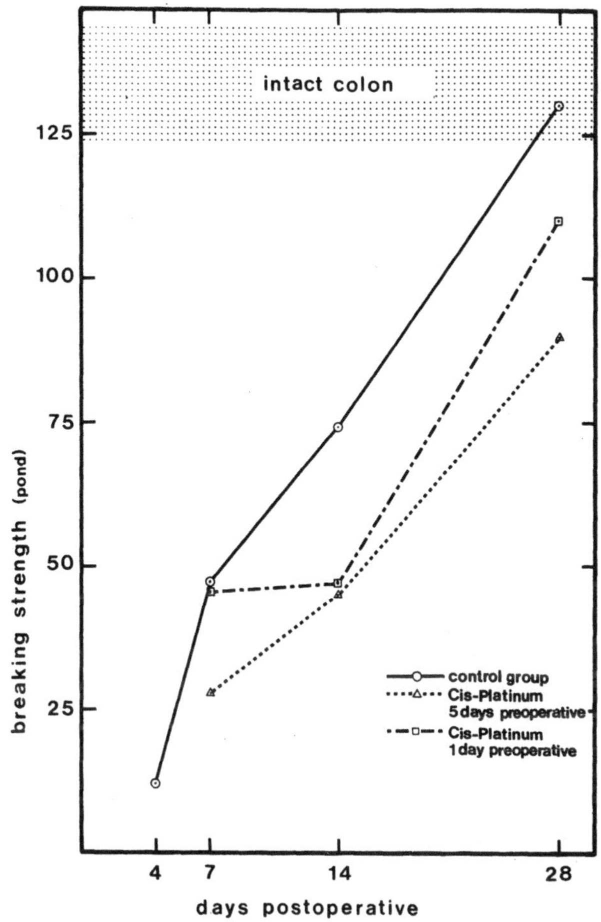

Fig. 2. WBS in the large-bowel anastomoses

received *cis*-platinum on day −5 preoperatively developed a WBS that was markedly lower. Again the most pronounced difference was noted on day +14, where the treatment groups had values of about 45 lb and the control group had values of about 74 lb. After 28 days, values in the control animals were normal, while those in the treatment groups were not quite normal.

Macroscopic and Light-Microscopic Findings

In the large-bowel anastomoses in the control group substantial amounts of connective tissue and scarred protuberances which produced adhesions to the neighboring loops were seen 7 days after surgery. In the treated animals, scar tissue in the area of the anastomoses was less evident and adhesions were fewer. The luminal surface showed the anastomoses and the connective tissue, and again the treated animals had less scar tissue.

In a histological section (Fig. 3a) of a nontreated large-bowel anastomosis after 14 days the connective tissue with marked protuberances is very clearly seen; in a large-bowel anastomosis treated with *cis*-platinum (Fig. 3b) the scar tissue is much less developed after 14 days and no protuberances are visible.

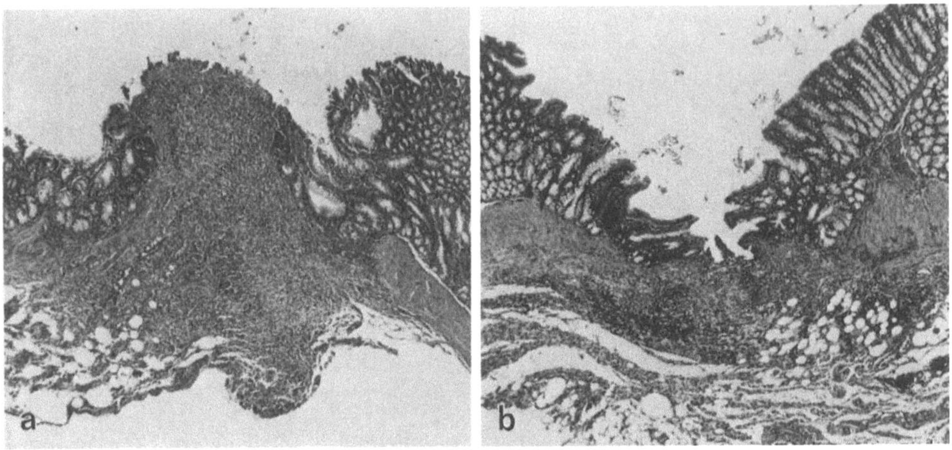

Fig. 3a, b. Longitudinal section of an untreated colon anastomosis (**a**) on day 14 after surgery and a section of a colon anastomosis of an animal treated preoperatively with *cis*-platinum (**b**). (H & E, 10×)

A similar picture is seen in the small-bowel anastomoses. The amount of scar tissue produced is lower in the treatment groups than in the control group, and there seem to be fewer fibers and more cellular elements in the treated anastomoses than in the untreated ones.

Microangiographically there is a delay in the growth of capillaries and vessels. On the 7th postoperative day the vessels have almost disappeared in the control anastomosis, whereas in the treatment group many parallel vessels can still be seen in the anastomosis.

Conclusion

Our study shows that *cis*-platinum has reduced WBS in rat bowel anastomoses when given preoperatively, by inhibiting connective tissue formation and delaying capillarization (Engelmann et al. 1983). As a result, we have stopped perioperative treatment with *cis*-platinum in cystectomy patients and we feel that before this drug can be used clinically as a perioperative adjuvant chemotherapy for bladder carcinoma further studies should be performed to determine the specific side-effects associated with surgery itself. We have initiated further studies concerning dosage and intervals of administration in connection with surgery, and also comparative trials with other drugs.

References

Engelmann U, Grimm K, Gröninger J, Bürger R, Jacobi GH (1983) Influence of *cis*-platinum on healing of enterostomies in the rat. Eur Urol 9: 45–49

Merrin C (1981) Adjuvant post-surgical chemotherapy with cyclophosphamide, doxorubicin hydrochloride and *cis*-diammine dichloroplatinum in patients with bladder cancer. In: Oliver, Hendry, Bloom (eds) Bladder cancer. Principles of combination therapy. Butterworths, London

Shamberger RC, Devereux DF, Brennan, MF (1981) The effect of chemotherapeutic agents on wound healing. Int Adv Surg Oncol 4: 15–58

Yagoda A (1979) Phase II trials with cis-dichlorodiammine-platinum (II) in the treatment of urothelial cancer. Cancer Treat Rep 63: 1565–1972

Drug Selection for Perioperative Chemotherapy

V. Hofmann, M. Berens, and G. Martz

Abteilung für Onkologie, Department für Innere Medizin, Universitätsspital Zürich, Rämistrasse 100, 8091 Zürich, Switzerland

Introduction

The purpose of chemotherapy delivered perioperatively (adjuvant treatment) is to destroy micrometastases that have spread beyond the primary tumor. There is no method that allows detection of small disseminated foci at this stage. Therefore, patients who are potentially tumor free after resection of the primary tumor will receive cytotoxic substances needlessly.

Up to now, anticancer substances that have been shown to be active in advanced disease have been used for adjuvant purposes. The effects of chemotherapy against measurable (advanced) disease are estimated by the reduction in size of tumor nodules and prolongation of survival. In contrast, the value of perioperative chemotherapy can only be estimated by its capacity to prolong disease-free and overall survival. It is therefore reasonable to assume that if few patients benefit from perioperative chemotherapy the statistical demonstration of its effect might be overlooked.

Ideally, treatment of patients who may harbor micrometastases should be tailored according to the drug sensitivity of primary tumor cells. Such an approach would avoid useless treatment of patients with resistant tumors and optimize the use of the most active substances. The best use of established agents on a rational basis is especially important since potent new drugs are developed only at a slow pace.

The recently developed clonogenic assay for in vitro culture of malignant cells has been shown to be of predictive value for drug sensitivity in retrospective correlation studies (Salmon et al. 1980; von Hoff et al. 1981a). In contrast to other predictive tests, the clonogenic assay measures the effect of drugs on the cell compartment that has been claimed to be responsible for tumor cell proliferation, i.e., the stem cell compartment (Selby et al. 1983).

Selection of Tumors for Drug Testing

Initial consideration should be given to determination of the tumor types for which drug sensitivity testing can provide useful and meaningful information. So far, experience with chemotherapy in large cohorts of patients has taught us that, depending on the tumor type, there is a broad range of clinical responses with variable impact on patient survival. At one end of the spectrum (Table 1) we find a small group of tumors that are highly responsive to

Recent Results in Cancer Research. Vol. 98

Table 1. Tumor types according to clinical response rate and probability of cure

Category	Response rate (%)	Cure (%)	Examples
I	> 70	> 50	Testicular carcinomas, Hodgkin's disease
II	> 70	< 20	Small cell carcinoma of lung, ovarian and breast carcinomas
III	< 30–40	0 (?)	Non-small cell lung cancer, malignant melanoma, colorectal carcinoma

chemotherapy, e.g., testicular carcinomas and Hodgkin's lymphomas; for this category of neoplasms, where induction of a complete remission by anticancer treatment is frequent and often synonymous with definitive cure, the use of cytotoxic agents at an early stage is debatable, since salvage treatment is highly effective even in advanced disease. Prognostic factors of early relapse would be more important than a test for drug sensitivity to improve the clinical outcome. A second, larger group of tumors can be classified as highly responsive to chemotherapy. However, even frequent complete remissions are of relatively short duration, and cure is thus rarely achieved. Small cell carcinomas of the lung and ovarian and breast carcinomas are good examples of this category. Thirdly, at the other end of the spectrum are mostly refractory tumors, for which cure is unlikely and reduction of tumor mass rare, e.g., melanomas and non-small cell lung and colorectal cancers. It is conceivable that patients with tumors from the second and third group would benefit most from in vitro drug sensitivity testing.

Prerequisites for Successful Drug Testing

Having defined tumor types for which in vitro drug testing would be of benefit, let us examine whether an in vitro test such as the clonogenic assay described above can be used to this end.

In the version developed by Hamburger and Salmon (1977), fresh tumor biopsies are prepared into single-cell suspensions. Aliquots of 1.5×10^6 cells are incubated with several drugs at different concentrations and washed, after which cultures are initiated in semisolid media. Formation of tumor colonies exposed to anticancer agents is compared with that in untreated controls.

Experience has shown that although the procedure appears simple, several problems can limit its use: in particular, the number of cells obtained after tumor disaggregation, the difficulty in preparing single-cell suspensions, and the number of samples with poor in vitro growth (Table 2).

Cell Numbers. Tumors may be very small and must be shared with the pathologist and frequently with other investigators (e.g., for determination of estrogen and progesterone receptor content in breast tumor samples). Since an in vitro drug test requires 1.5×10^6 cells/drug concentration, small specimens frequently yield cell numbers that do not allow testing of a sufficient number of drugs, which would be particularly important for refractory

Table 2. Requirements and limitations of successful in vitro drug testing

Requirements	Limitations
Sample size (total cell number)	Testing of few drugs
Single-cell suspensions	Clumps and reaggregated single cells bias final scoring
> 70% of samples with > 30 colonies per dish (better > 100 colonies)	Most tumors produce few colonies

tumors. In the search for an active substance, the probability of finding an effective agent is greater if a large number of drugs is tested for efficacy.

Single-Cell Suspensions. The preparation of a single-cell suspension is crucial, since the assay is designed to detect colony formation that should originate only from single cells following multiple divisions. Frequently, disaggregation techniques are unable to eliminate small clumps or to yield a sufficient cell number, even from relatively large tumor specimens. Clumps persisting in the final suspensions can introduce substantial bias in the final scoring of the plates.

Cloning Efficiency. A fundamental aspect of the assay is related to its capacity to promote growth. In this context we will not consider biological factors that affect growth, such as cell-cell interactions, conditioned media, growth factors, etc. (Steele 1977), but rather simply analyze the performance of the assay based on published reports and personal experience. For evaluation of the inhibitory effect of drugs a minimum of 20–30 colonies per control has been recommended (von Hoff et al. 1981a), which corresponds to a plating efficiency of 0.006%, defined as number of colonies per plated cells. The cloning efficiency represents the same number of colonies related to the number of tumor cells in the plated suspensions.

Some authors do not report on samples with insufficient growth to allow drug testing. Most investigators indicate the number of samples that provided any clonal growth, which gives the impression that the assay is applicable for drug testing of most tumors (Hamburger and Salmon 1977; Buick et al. 1980). The first report on a large group of tumors that was analyzed by both criteria, i.e., by any growth and by adequate growth for drug testing, was published by von Hoff et al. (1981a). Out of 800 various tumors, only 199 (25%) were evaluable for drug sensitivity assays, but about 60% showed some growth. A subsequent analysis of 8000 tumors confirmed that only 31% had sufficient growth for drug testing (von Hoff 1983). In our own experience with 204 tumors processed between July 1980 and June 1981, some growth was found in 74%, but drug testing was possible in only 32% of tumor specimens (Hofmann, unpublished data). Such an analysis does not reveal the importance of histological subtypes and the origin of tumor biopsies (malignant effusion versus solid biopsies). We have consistently observed that tumor cells isolated from effusions show higher success rates (49%) than solid specimens (27%). This has also been reported by other authors (Salmon 1980; Sandbach et al. 1982). It also appears that most "cloning" laboratories are successful with some tumor types: ovarian carcinomas, malignant melanomas, neuroblastomas, and multiple myelomas. Despite worldwide use of the assay there is still a lack of published reports noting precise success rates by sample size, tumor type, and specimen origin. Table 3 gives a partial presentation of the experience of several groups with regard to the tumor types that would be of importance in an adjuvant setting. Some growth was reported in 43%–90% of a varied collection of histological subtypes. Adequate growth allowing drug testing was described for 45%–73% of tumors. These values are probably too optimistic if it is borne in mind that drug testing would be performed solely on primary tumors, which have lower plating efficiencies than metastases (especially effusions) and also yield low cell numbers.

For these reasons, the in vitro clonogenic assay cannot be expected to provide drug sensitivity results for more than 30% of all tumors. However, some tumor types, especially ovarian adenocarcinoma and malignant melanoma, appear to grow with the highest success rates and could, therefore, be considered for in vitro studies in parallel with clinical trials.

Clinical Interpretation of In Vitro Results

Retrospective studies have shown that inhibition of tumor colony formation by at least 70% with clinically achievable doses of a given drug is correlated with an objective response to the same substance given in vivo (Salmon et al. 1980; von Hoff et al. 1981a). Thus far, patients with sensitive tumors in vitro have experienced only short remissions.

Table 3. Analysis of cloning success in different laboratories

Cloning success (%)				
Category	Examples	≥ 5 Colonies	≥ 30 Colonies	Reference
II	Lung, small cell	38/61 (62)		von Hoff et al. (1981a)
		32/36 (89)		Carney et al. (1981)
	Ovarian	22/27 (81)		Ozols et al. (1980)
		53/71 (75)		von Hoff et al. (1981a)
		26/31 (84)		Hamburger et al. (1980)
		21/25 (84)	16/25 (64)	Hofmann, unpublished data
	Breast	160/225 (71)	102/225 (45)	Sandbach et al. (1982)
III	Lung, non-small cell	45/75 (60)		von Hoff et al. (1981b)
	Malignant melanoma	64/93 (69)	51/93 (55)	von Hoff et al. (1982)
			16/22 (73)	Pavelic et al. (1980)
		22/38 (58)		Meyskens (1980)
	Colorectal		8/11 (73)	Pavelic et al. (1980)
		28/38 (74)		von Hoff et al. (1981a)
		3/7 (43)		Buick et al. (1980)
	Renal	45/50 (90)	32/50 (64)	Sarosdy et al. (1982)

Consequently, the reduction of colony number by only 70% may leave a resistant subpopulation that causes rapid regrowth of the tumor after subcurative therapy. Since the intent of perioperative chemotherapy is to destroy the last surviving tumor cell, drugs, or combinations of several compounds, might be expected to prevent all single cells from forming colonies in vitro. However, this degree of in vitro cell kill will be inaccurately measured if control plates grow only 30 colonies. Detection of 95%–100% colony inhibition with a reasonable degree of certainty would require higher plating efficiencies in control plates. For example, a drug showing 95% inhibition would leave 5 colonies when control plates contain 100 colonies. Such precise determinations would be possible for few tumor specimens. With control dishes of only 30 colonies, for the same degree of drug-inhibitory activity less than 2 colonies would have to be detected. Several technical reasons, such as persistent clumps, reproducibility of the assay, and the optical characteristics of the plates, prevent this level of accuracy. These considerations indicate that possibly even fewer tumor samples than suggested above would be adequate for selection of perioperative chemotherapy.

One additional aspect that deserves careful evaluation is the fact that the true-positive rate of the assay for an individual patient is dependent on the therapeutic response rate of the tumor category (Table 1). The true-positive rate (TPR) indicates the probability that the test will correctly predict drug sensitivity and is defined by:

$$\mathrm{TPR} = \frac{\text{Number of responding patients with test indicating sensitivity (true-positive test)}}{\text{True-positive tests + tests falsely indicating sensitivity (false-positive test)}}\,.$$

This equation shows that the number of false-positive tests influences the true-positive rate. It must be recognized that the number of false-positive tests will rise with increasing clinical resistance of the tumor types to chemotherapy. This can be illustrated by the following example. Assuming that the performance of the assay (i.e., sensitivity and specificity) remains constant regardless of the therapeutic response rate of the tumor, a correct prediction is possible for about 90% of patients suffering from a tumor that has a clinical response rate of 50%. This value drops to 40% for a tumor with only 10% likelihood of clinical response. In other words, in the presence of highly refractory tumors, when the in vitro test indicates that the tumor is responsive to a given drug, at best only 40% of the patients found to be sensitive in vitro can potentially benefit from this information. Since better treatment is urgently needed for this category of tumors, the use of an in vitro assay will be of marginal benefit for this purpose. For a tumor like malignant melanoma, although it grows with a high success rate, the in vitro results will not significantly improve therapeutic outcome.

Summary

A wide variety of tumor types can be successfully grown with the clonogenic assay. However, few tumor types perform adequately for routine drug sensitivity testing, e.g., ovarian carcinoma and malignant melanoma. Because of insufficient in vitro growth, the cloning system cannot help substantially in indicating active substances for epidemiologically frequent tumors that usually have a poor prognosis, such as colorectal cancers and non-small cell lung and breast cancers.

The degree of in vitro cell kill that would correspond to complete eradication of micrometastases is unknown. The identification of individual patients sensitive to a given antineoplastic agent becomes more difficult as the tumor becomes more refractory to treatment.

At this moment, the clonogenic assay appears most promising for trials dealing with the treatment of ovarian adenocarcinoma.

References

Buick RN, Fry SE, Salmon SE (1980) Application of in vitro soft agar techniques for growth of tumor cells to study of colon cancer. Cancer 45: 1238–1242

Carney DN, Gazdor AF, Bunn PA Jr, Minna JD (1981) In vitro cloning of small cell carcinoma of the lung. In: Gaco FA, Oldham RK, Bunn PA Jr (eds) Small cell lung cancer. Grune and Stratton, New York, pp 79–94

Hamburger AW, Salmon SE (1977) Primary bioassay of human tumor stem cells. Science 197: 461–463

Hamburger AW, Salmon SE, Alberts DS (1980) Development of a bioassay for ovarian carcinoma colony-forming cells. In: Salmon SE (ed) Cloning of human tumor stem cells. Liss, New York, pp 63–73 (Progress in clinical and biological research, vol 48)

Meyskens FL Jr (1980) Human melanoma colony formation in soft agar. In: Salmon SE (ed) Cloning of human tumor stem cells. Liss, New York, pp 85–99 (Progress in clinical and biological research, vol 48)

Ozols RF, Willson JKV, Grotzinger KR, Young RC (1980) Cloning of human ovarian cancer cells in soft agar from malignant effusions and peritoneal washings. Cancer Res 40: 2743–2747

Pavelic ZP, Slocum HK, Rustum YM, Creaven PJ, Nowak NJ, Karakousis C, Takita H, Mittelman A (1980) Growth of cell colonies in soft agar from biopsies of different solid tumors. Cancer Res 40: 4151–4158

Salmon SE (1980) Cloning of human tumor stem cells. Liss, New York (Progress in clinical and biological research, vol 48)

Salmon SE, Alberts DS, Durie BGM, Meyskens FL, Jones SE, Soehnlen B, Chen H-SG, Moon T (1980) Clinical correlations of drug sensitivity in the human tumor stem cell assay. Recent Results Cancer Res 74: 300–305

Sandbach J, von Hoff DD, Clark G, Cruz AB Jr, Obrien M (1982) Direct cloning of human breast cancer in soft agar culture. Cancer 50: 1315–1321

Sarosdy MF, Lamm DL, Radwin HM, von Hoff DD (1982) Clonogenic assay and in vitro chemosensitivity testing of human urologic malignancies. Cancer 50: 1332–1338

Selby P, Buick RN, Tarmock I (1983) A critical appraisal of the "human tumor stem cell assay." N Engl J Med 308: 129–133

Steele GG (1977) Growth kinetics of tumors: cell population kinetics in relation of the growth and treatment of cancer. Clarendon, Oxford

von Hoff DD (1983) Send this patient's tumor for culture and sensitivity. N Engl J Med 308: 154–155

von Hoff DD, Casper J, Bradley E, Sandbach J, Jones D, Makuch R (1981a) Association between human tumor colony-forming assay results and response of an individual patient's tumor to chemotherapy. Am J Med 70: 1027–1032

von Hoff DD, Weisenthal LM, Ihde DC, Mathews MJ, Layard M, Makuch R (1981b) Growth of lung cancer colonies from bronchoscopy washings. Cancer 48: 400–403

von Hoff DD, Forseth B, Mitelmann HR, Harris G, Rowan S, Coltman CA Jr (1982) Direct cloning of human malignant melanoma in soft agar culture. Cancer 50: 696–701

Techniques for Avoiding Surgical Complications in Chemotherapy-Treated Cancer Patients

J. H. Raaf

Cleveland Clinic Cancer Center,
9500 Euclid Avenue, Cleveland, OH 44106, USA

Introduction

With the development of more effective antineoplastic drugs for the treatment of solid malignant tumors, the use of systemic chemotherapy in the perioperative period has become increasingly attractive. Strategies have evolved for administering chemotherapy *pre*operatively to render large tumors more easily resected, *intra*operatively in isolation-perfusion systems (often in combination with hyperthermia), and *post*operatively as an adjuvant or to treat residual disease. It is possible, however, that the benefits of perioperative chemotherapy may be offset by an increase in the incidence of complications, particularly with respect to wound healing. The well-known toxic effects of chemotherapeutic agents on actively replicating normal cells suggest that antineoplastic drugs could easily lead to wound problems such as infection or dehiscence.

Laboratory studies in which chemotherapeutic agents are given to experimental animals in the pre-, intra-, or postoperative period have not been reassuring, since significant impairment of wound healing by these drugs has been demonstrated. Results published in the 1950s and 1960s varied, because experimental designs were dissimilar. When nitrogen mustard (Farhat et al. 1958; Hardesty 1958), thio-TEPA (Conn et al. 1957; Pisesky et al. 1959; Rath and Enquiest 1959), or 5-fluorouracil (Staley et al. 1961; Goldman et al. 1969) was administered as a single agent in the perioperative period, results varying from no effect to marked impairment were recorded. More recent, well-controlled animal studies with Adriamycin have documented very significant delays in the development of tensile strength after wounding (Devereux et al. 1979; Shamberger et al. 1981). However, a vast clinical experience in surgical adjuvant trials in man suggests that postoperative adjuvant chemotherapy has almost no practical deleterious effect on wound healing in the clinical setting. Of course, in most cases the adjuvant drugs were started after the initial phases of wound healing were complete.

A well-standardized experimental technique was developed by Cohen et al. (1975a, b). Using measurements of wound breaking strength in chemotherapy-treated mice, these investigators compared the effects on wound healing of various antineoplastic agents delivered IP at therapeutic levels. Quantitative decreases in strength were shown, but no significant wound complications were seen in the mice and the superficial wound infection rate was less than 1%. Therefore, though they found that many antitumor drugs (vincristine, methotrexate, dactinomycin, BCNU, cyclophosphamide, and bleomycin) have a diverse range of measurable effects at different phases of the healing process,

Recent Results in Cancer Research. Vol. 98

clinically successful healing proceeded in all cases, and none of the drugs tested caused wound disruption in the intact animals.

Pre- and Intraoperative Chemotherapy

Several trials have now been conducted to determine whether patients with solid malignant tumors can benefit from preoperative chemotherapy. The results have been encouraging, since a decrease in gross tumor size and histological evidence for drug-induced tumor necrosis have been seen. Rosen et al. (1982) have used high-dose methotrexate and citrovorum factor rescue, plus the combination bleomycin, cyclophosphamide, and dactinomycin, in patients with osteogenic sarcoma. Patients who did not respond to this combination of preoperative chemotherapy were changed postoperatively from methotrexate to *cis*-platinum and Adriamycin.

Kelsen et al. (1982) claim increased resectability in patients with esophageal carcinoma following preoperative cisplatin, vindesine, and bleomycin. Morton et al. (1976) managed patients with extremity skeletal and soft-tissue sarcomas using preoperative intra-arterial Adriamycin plus radiation therapy, claiming increased frequency of salvage of a functional extremity. Favorable results have also been reported by Calvo et al. (1980), who treated patients with regionally confined solid tumors with intra-arterial cisplatin. This approach may be useful in patients with pelvic sarcomas, to make hemipelvectomy more feasible.

At the present time, intraoperative chemotherapy refers to attempts at "regional chemotherapy", the selective delivery of an antineoplastic agent to a specific anatomical area. Methods of regional chemotherapy include: (a) continuous arterial infusion; (b) tourniquet (bolus) infusion, and (c) isolation-perfusion (usually in combination with hyperthermia). These methods all depend on cannulation of a specific artery and can theoretically result in a high tissue level of the drug(s) with reduced systemic toxicity compared with conventional peripheral IV administration. Experience is limited so far, though encouraging results have been reported by McBride et al. (1981) with isolation-perfusion used both prophylactically and therapeutically for melanoma and by Karakousis (1979), who has developed the simpler tourniquet infusion method. Complications resulting from the instillation of very high doses of drugs into an extremity can be serious, and amputations have been required as a result. Thus investigational work in this area must be intelligently controlled and patients carefully selected.

Postoperative (Adjuvant) Chemotherapy

Advances in medical oncology have led to increased use of potent and effective chemotherapeutic agents as adjuvants in an attempt to increase patient survival. When the tumor burden has been reduced by surgery, chemotherapy can then theoretically be more effective. Oncologists may be reluctant to initiate aggressive systemic chemotherapy in the immediate postoperative period for fear of catastrophic complications such as wound infection, wound dehiscence, or anastomotic breakdown. The surgeon may retain vivid memories of poor wound healing in a patient debilitated by an advanced tumor. However, no adjuvant trial to date has reported significant impairment to healing of the wound.

Unfortunately, most clinical reports lack detailed information on wounds or the timing of the administration of drugs relative to the surgery. Thus evaluation of different drugs, combinations, and dosages is difficult. Chemotherapy in most studies was not begun until 2–4 weeks after the surgical procedures, by which time a surgical wound is essentially healed. In these reports wound complications are said to be minimal. Examples are the studies of adjuvant thio-TEPA for breast cancer (Donegan 1974), dactinomycin for Wilm's tumor (Fernback and Martyn 1966), mitomycin C for gastric carcinoma (Hattori et al. 1966), 5-fluorouracil for colon cancer (Higgins et al. 1971), cyclophosphamide and methotrexate for lung carcinoma (Shields et al. 1977), hexamethylmelamine and 5-fluorouracil in patients with ovarian cancer (Kardinal and Luce 1977), and chlorambucil, methotrexate, and dactinomycin for testicular cancer (Ansfield et al. 1969). Thus adjuvant chemotherapy appears to have little clinically important effect on wound healing. This is in striking contrast to other factors which clearly *do* affect wound healing, for example previous radiation therapy, heavy pretreatment with steroids, presence of sepsis, or malnutrition.

In view of our clinical observations to date and our present understanding of the mechanisms and extent to which drugs may alter the normal healing process, we conclude there is no contraindication to the use of perioperative chemotherapy in well-planned protocols. The potential benefit of destroying residual microscopic malignant disease in the adjuvant setting is a particularly acceptable risk when weighed against the minimal likelihood of wound complications.

Vascular Access Procedures in Cancer Patients

Recently attention has been focused on the methodology of chemotherapy administration, and this field has become almost as specialized as that of vascular access in patients with renal failure who receive hemodialysis. Cancer patients with poor peripheral surface veins suffer the discomfort of multiple (often unsuccessful) venipunctures. As inpatients they may be at high risk from the complications of central line insertion, which can be fatal if hemothorax occurs in association with chemotherapy- or disease-related thrombocytopenia. Extravasation of chemotherapeutic drugs is another danger, which can result in significant soft tissue loss if the agent is Adriamycin (Larson 1982) or mitomycin C (Argenta and Manders 1983).

It is our opinion that special methods for establishing safe vascular access are required in high-risk cancer patients with thrombocytopenia, susceptibility to infection, or nutritional debility (Raaf 1984a). We perform two types of access procedures: insertion of long-term silastic right atrial catheters, and placement of polytetrafluoroethylene (PTFE) arteriovenous vascular access grafts. Both procedures are done under local anesthesia (except in young children), using a strict sterile technique. Long-term silastic right atrial catheters are inserted via the internal or external jugular vein. A 2.2 mm OD Broviac catheter is placed in children, and a 3.2 mm OD Hickman catheter in adults. The cephalic vein is seldom used since it often has been sclerosed by previous chemotherapy. A fine intestinal probe is used during the tunneling step, to decrease trauma and hemorrhage. Leukemic and bone marrow transplant patients receive either two simultaneous Broviac catheters placed through separate, parallel tunnels and venotomies into the right internal jugular vein (Raaf 1984b), or a new dual lumen silastic catheter (Quinton Instrument Co.). This provides one route of access for parenteral nutrition, which most of the these patients require, and a second port for blood products and all other medications as well as a channel through which to obtain blood samples.

During placement of a silastic catheter, venotomy leakage is prevented by a 5–0 polyproplylene pursestring suture. A single absorbable 4–0 polyglycolic acid suture at the skin exit secures the catheter and prevents dislodgement before the Dacron cuff becomes firmly fixed. Correct positioning of the tip of the catheter(s) in the right atrium is always confirmed by fluoroscopy before the patient leaves the operating room. Percutaneous catheter placement using a peel-away pacemaker wire introducer sheath is possible in selected patients, but generally we prefer an open technique. Individuals with superior vena cava syndrome receive a silastic catheter introduced through the femoral vein, with the tip positioned in the inferior vena cava at L3. Patients with low platelet counts are infused intra- or postoperatively if required to control hemorrhage, but not on a routine preoperative basis.

After placement of a long-term silastic catheter, chemotherapy is often started the same day. Nonetheless, the overall complication rate in 280 patients has been acceptable, about 21%, including minor problems such as temporary postoperative bleeding requiring a pressure dressing, exit site erythema, suspected catheter sepsis, and catheter damage during dressing changes. This is despite the fact that 44% of these patients have leukemia or are bone marrow transplant recipients and many of them have severe neutropenia (< 1,000 WBC/mm^3) or thrombocytopenia (< 20,000 platelets/mm^3). Pneumo- or hemothorax was not encountered, and there was no mortality associated with catheter placement. Cervical wound infections following catheter placement have been extremely rare: only 1 wound infection (0.4%) and 1 nonhealing wound (in an irradiated patient with mycosis fungoides).

In selected individuals who are to receive adjuvant chemotherapy we have placed PTFE vascular access grafts (6 mm) in the upper arm, end-to-side to the brachial artery and the axillary vein (Raaf 1979, 1980). A femoral artery-to-femoral vein loop graft is a satisfactory alternative. The advantage of these grafts is the lack of need for maintenance care when not in use. Therefore, PTFE grafts are most useful in patients receiving outpatient chemotherapy, but continuous inpatient IV infusion is possible by percutaneous placement of an 18 gauge plastic cannula into the graft (Raaf and Ennis 1982). The complication rate is higher for the PTFE grafts than for silastic catheters. Of 53 grafts, 19 eventually thrombosed and required revision, though only 2 became infected (overall complication rate of 40%); and 5 of the 53 grafts were eventually removed. Our current preference is to use silastic catheters in most patients, because of the ease of insertion and removal.

Clinical Guidelines for Avoiding Complications

For a variety of reasons, patients who have received chemotherapy may become candidates for a surgical procedure. The surgeon and anesthesiologist must review the patient's history with respect to the agents received, to avoid predictable complications (Table 1). Obviously surgery should be avoided during periods of drug-induced pancytopenia except in emergency circumstances. Special precautions are advisable if the patient has received certain drugs. Patients treated with bleomycin should not be given high oxygen concentrations during anesthesia, due to the increased danger of pulmonary oxygen toxicity. Recipients of Adriamycin should have careful evaluation and monitoring of cardiac function. Renal failure is avoided in cisplatin-treated patients by prehydration and mannitol. Halothane is not used, to avoid confusion with hepatic failure caused by hepatic

Table 1. Postoperative complications to be avoided in chemotherapy-treated patients

Complication	Agent	Cause
1. Infection	Many	Neutropenia
2. Hemorrhage	Many	Thrombocytopenia
3. Renal failure	*cis*-Platinum	Renal toxicity (prehydrate)
4. Respiratory failure	Bleomycin	Oxygen toxicity (avoid high pO_2)
5. Congestive failure	Adriamycin	Cardiomyopathy (limit dose)
6. Liver failure	Halothane	Hepatitis (use other anesthetics)

metastases Meticulous surgical technique is essential in steroid-treated patients. In malnourished cancer patients, wound disruption can be avoided by use of parenteral nutrition.

Often the surgeon and medical oncologist must decide together when to begin chemotherapy in a patient who has just undergone a surgical procedure. For the reasons described above, there is no need to fear that chemotherapy will interfere with healing of the surgical wound. Obviously if the surgeon anticipates that a patient will receive chemotherapy postoperatively, the wound should be closed in the manner considered most secure. We use nonabsorbable sutures for the fascial closure, and we often place heavy nylon "retention" sutures through all layers of the abdominal wall (Fig. 1) by the method of Smead as described by Jones et al. (1941). In a patient with very extensive tumor, poor nutrition, or high risk for infection, the abdominal incision can be closed in one layer using No. 2 monofilament nylon and a double-loop mass closure technique (Karakousis 1980). These mass closure methods provide protection against dehiscence if a wound infection occurs (Malt 1977). Sutures are left in place for at least 3 weeks. Wound healing may be

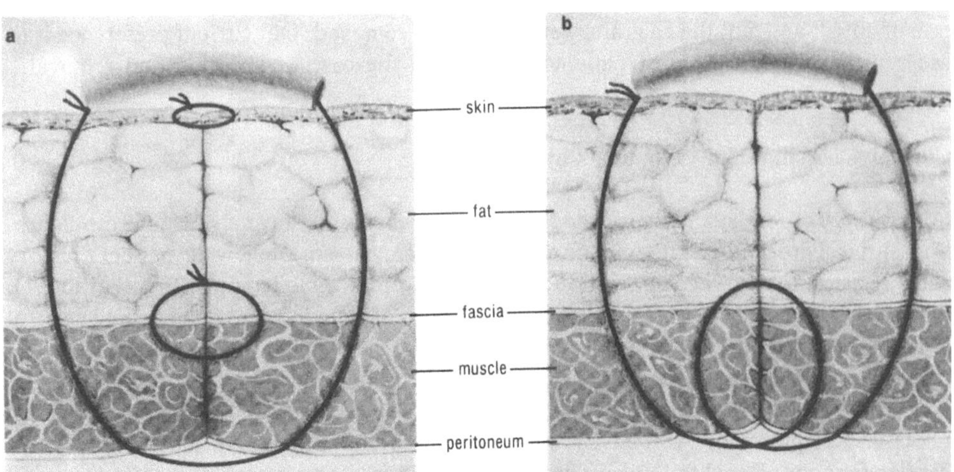

Fig. 1. a No. 2 nylon retention suture; **b** No. 2 nylon double-loop mass suture

Table 2. Steps to improve wound healing in patients receiving perioperative chemotherapy

1. Meticulous surgical technique (e.g., nylon retention sutures)
2. Careful skin preparation and liberal antibiotic coverage
3. Parenteral nutrition in malnourished patients
4. After a major procedure (laparotomy, thoracotomy, major amputation), interval of 7–10 days before start chemotherapy

promoted in a poorly nourished patient by giving pre- and postoperative parenteral alimentation. This is particularly indicated if an extended period of anorexia is anticipated as a side-effect of chemotherapy.

Chemotherapy should not be started before the initial phase of wound healing is complete and the period of high risk for developing a serious complication of surgery has passed (Ferguson 1982). For a simple lymph node biopsy this may be only a few days. After laparotomy, thoracotomy, or radical soft tissue resection it is usually 7–10 days. It would obviously be more difficult to control a serious wound infection or hemorrhage in a patient who is pancytopenic due to drug-induced bone marrow depression. Also, there is little theoretical advantage to starting adjuvant chemotherapy during the first postoperative 7–10 days. This interval allows the patient to become ambulatory, clear any atelectasis, and advance to a regular diet. Drains and catheters can be removed. There are exceptions where chemotherapy may be urgently needed, such as in individuals whose laparotomy reveals extensive lymphoma. In these patients it is reasonable to proceed with appropriate chemotherapy as soon as the patient is hemodynamically stable.

References

Ansfield FL, Korbitz BC, Davis HL, Raminez G (1969) Triple drug therapy in testicular tumors. Cancer 24: 442–446

Argenta LC, Manders EK (1983) Mitomycin C extravasation injuries. Cancer 51: 1080–1082

Calvo DB, Patt YZ, Wallace S, Chuang VP, Benjamin RS, Pritchard JD, Hersh EM, Bodey GP Sr, Mariglit GM (1980) Phase I–II trial of percutaneous intra-arterial cis-diamminedichloro platinum (II) for regionally confined malignancy. Cancer 45: 1278–1283

Cohen SC, Gabelnick HL, Johnson RK, Goldin A (1975a) Effects of antineoplastic agents on wound healing in mice. Surgery 78: 238–244

Cohen SC, Gabelnick HL, Johnson RK, Goldin A (1975b) Effects of cyclophosphamide and Adriamycin on the healing of surgical wounds in mice. Cancer 36: 1277–1281

Conn JH, Leb SM, Hardy JD (1957) Effect of nitrogen mustard and thio-TEPA on wound healing. Surg Forum 8: 80–83

Devereux DF, Thibault L, Boretos J, Brennan MF (1979) The quantitative and qualitative impairment of wound healing by Adriamycin. Cancer 43: 932–938

Donegan WL (1974) Extended surgical adjuvant thio-TEPA for mammary carcinoma. Arch Surg 109: 187–192

Farhat SM, Amer NS, Weeks DS, Musselman MM (1958) Effect of mechlorethamine hydrochloride (nitrogen mustard) on healing of abdominal wounds. Arch Surg 76: 749–753

Ferguson MK (1982) The effect of antineoplastic agents on wound healing. Surg Gynecol Obstet 154: 421–429

Fernback DJ, Martyn DT (1966) Role of dactinomycin on the improved survival of children with Wilm's tumor. JAMA 195: 1005–1009

Goldman LI, Lowe S, Al-Saleem T (1969) Effect of fluorouracil on intestinal anastomoses in the rat. Arch Surg 98: 303–304

Hardesty WH (1958) The effect of cytotoxic drugs on wound healing in rats. Cancer Res 18:581–584

Hattori T, Ito I, Hirata K, Iizuka T, Abe K (1966) Results of combined treatment in patients with cancer of the stomach: palliative gastrectomy, large-dose mitomycin-C, and bone marrow transplantation. Gan 57:441–451

Higgins GA, Dwight RW, Smith JV, Keehn RJ (1971) Fluorouracil as an adjuvant to surgery in carcinoma of the colon. Arch Surg 102:339–343

Jones TE, Newell ET, Brubaker RE (1941) The use of alloy steel wire in the closure of abdominal wounds. Surg Gynecol Obstet 72:1056–1059

Karakousis CP (1979) Tourniquet infusion chemotherapy in extremities with malignant lesions. Surg Gynecol Obstet 149:481–490

Karakousis CP (1980) One layer closure of the abdominal wall. Surg Gynecol Obstet 150:243–244

Kardinal CG, Luce JK (1977) Evaluation of a hexamethylmelamine and 5-fluorouracil combination in the treatment of advanced ovarian carcinoma. Cancer Treat Rep 61:1691–1693

Kelsen DP, Bains M, Hilaris B, Chapman R, McCormack P, Alexander T, Hopfan S, Martini N (1982) Combination chemotherapy of esophageal carcinoma using cisplatin, vindesine, and bleomycin. Cancer 49:1174–1177

Larson DL (1982) Treatment of tissue extravasation by antitumor agents. Cancer 49:1796–1782

Malt RA (1977) Abdominal incisions, sutures, and sacrilege. N Engl J Med 297:722–723

McBride CM, Smith JL, Brown BW (1981) Primary malignant melanoma of the limbs: a re-evaluation using microstaging techniques. Cancer 48:1463–1468

Morton DL, Eilber FR, Townsend CM, Grant TT, Mirra J, Weisenburger TH (1976) Limb salvage from a multidisciplinary treatment approach for skeletal and soft tissue sarcomas of the extremity. Ann Surg 184:268–278

Pisesky W, Williams HTG, MacKenzie WC (1959) The effect of triethylene thiophosphoramide (thio-TEPA) and 17-ethyl-19 nortestosterone (Nivelar) on wound healing. Can J Surg 2:291–294

Raaf JH (1979) Vascular access grafts for chemotherapy: use in forty patients at M.D. Anderson Hospital. Ann Surg 190:614–622

Raaf JH (1980) Vascular access prostheses in the management of cancer patients. Clin Bull 10:91–101

Raaf JH (1984a) Vascular access for chemotherapy. In: Waltzer WC (ed) Vascular Access Surgery chap 14. Grune and Stratton, New York, pp 161–192

Raaf JH (1984b) Two Broviac catheters for intensive long-term support of cancer patients. Surg Gynecol Obstet 158:173–176

Raaf JH, Ennis J (1982) Long-term percutaneous catheter inserted into a polytetrafluoroethylene graft for administration of chemotherapy. Arch Surg 117:514–515

Rath H, Enquist IF (1959) The effect of thio-TEPA on wound healing. Arch Surg 79:812–814

Rosen G, Caparros B, Huvos AG, Kosloff C, Nirenberg A, Cacavio A, Marcove R, Lane T, Mehta B, Urban C (1982) Preoperative chemotherapy for osteogenic sarcoma: selection of postoperative adjuvant chemotherapy based on the response of the primary tumor to preoperative chemotherapy. Cancer 49:1221–1230

Shamberger RC, Devereux DF, Brennan MF (1981) The effect of chemotherapeutic agents on wound healing. Int Adv Surg Oncol 4:15–58

Shields, TW, Humphrey EW, Eastridge CE, Keehn RJ (1977) Adjuvant cancer chemotherapy after resection of carcinoma of the lung. Cancer 40:2057–2062

Staley CJ, Trippel OH, Preston FW (1961) Influence of 5-fluorouracil on wound healing. Surgery 49:450–453

Methodological and Statistical Aspects in Perioperative Chemotherapy Trials

R. D. Gelber*

Department of Biostatistics, Dana-Farber Cancer Institute,
44 Binney Street, Boston, MA 02115, USA

Introduction

Historically, local regional treatment alone (with surgery or radiation therapy) has been the main approach to the management of patients with newly diagnosed cancer without evidence of distant metastases. Unfortunately, this form of primary therapy alone is not curative for a large number of patients. Failure is felt to be due in large part to the presence of micrometastatic disease that remains undetected at initial diagnosis. Thus, in an effort to destroy these micrometastases, chemotherapy has been introduced as an adjuvant to the primary treatment.

For the purpose of this discussion, surgery will be considered the primary treatment used. Although the term "adjuvant" means in addition to, our use of the term "adjuvant chemotherapy" has come to mean the administration of chemotherapy *following* surgery as primary treatment. Cytotoxic drugs are administered after primary therapy, but prior to evidence of metastatic failure or recurrence. Usually, drug administration is started within 4–8 weeks of the surgery. Technically, this form of adjuvant chemotherapy might be more accurately referred to as postoperative chemotherapy. Similar clarity can be achieved by defining the nature of adjuvant treatments according to the timing of drug administration relative to the surgical procedure. Specifically, preoperative chemotherapy is given before surgery, intraoperative chemotherapy is given during the operation and perioperative chemotherapy is given in the inmediate postoperative period. In each of these, chemotherapy is an integral part of the primary treatment program. It is given prior to recurrence or relapse, and is an adjuvant to the surgery. The crucial difference among these approaches is the timing of chemotherapy relative to the surgical procedure. Each approach has its own advantages and disadvantages in terms of patient management, ease of administration, evaluation potential, and theoretical biological justification. This presentation focuses on the statistical and methodological aspects of evaluating forms of adjuvant chemotherapy. In particular, the therapeutic evaluation in the usual adjuvant setting (postoperative chemotherapy) and the evaluation of the perioperative approach will be contrasted.

First, the similarities between the two settings will be discussed, with particular emphasis on the role of the controlled clinical trial and the need to study a large number of patients

---

* For the Ludwig Breast Cancer Study Group

Recent Results in Cancer Research. Vol. 98

followed for a prolonged period of time. Second, some of the major differences in terms of clinical trials considerations will be highlighted. The critical issue of timing of treatment, the fact that important information about eligibility and stratification factors may not be known at the time of patient entry, and the impact of having a patient population that is different from that encountered in the more usual adjuvant setting will be discussed. Finally, the importance of evaluating all patients in the analysis to yield unbiased results will be stressed as particularly relevant to the perioperative chemotherapy trial.

Similarities Between Conventional Adjuvant Trials and Perioperative Chemotherapy Trials

The methodology of the controlled clinical trial has been developed as the most convincing way to conduct comparative evaluations of cancer treatment programs (Byar 1979; Chalmers et al. 1972; Zelen 1983). Both trials of usual adjuvant therapy and those of perioperative chemotherapy must follow the guidelines for sound experimental design. A protocol document must be prepared to give a clear statement of the study objectives, patient population, patient registration, treatment administration, follow-up schedule, end-point evaluation and documentation, and sample size requirements.

The use of randomization as the mechanism for allocating treatments to patients is essential for conducting unbiased treatment comparisons. When each patient has the same opportunity of receiving any of the therapies under investigation, the characteristics of the different treatment groups will be "alike on average" with respect to all factors that are likely to affect outcome. In this way, any observed differences in results between groups will tend to be due to real differences in treatment effectiveness. Prospective randomization also guarantees that neither the physician nor the patient knows in advance which therapy will be assigned. This helps to eliminate both conscious and unconscious biases due to physician or patient selection. Prognostic features of the patients or the disease may effect the ultimate outcome far more than any real differences between therapies. Many such prognostic factors may be unknown or difficult to quantify. It is essential in any comparative treatment evaluation that observed differences attributed to treatment are, in fact, due to treatment and not to other factors which might bias the results. Thus, the use of randomization is an important feature of comparative trials regardless of the nature of the adjuvant therapy used.

Another similarity between the more usual adjuvant trials and perioperative chemotherapy trials is that both require large numbers of patients to ensure that moderate but important treatment differences will be detected. In many situations, establishing negative result may be as important as establishing that a treatment difference exists. The importance of sufficient sample size is discussed by several authors (cf. Freiman et al. 1978; Peto et al. 1976, 1977). According to Table 2 presented by Peto et al. (1976, p 610), approximately 100 failures per treatment must be observed at the time of an analysis for there to be an 80% chance of detecting a 50% difference in failure rates between two treatment programs. This treatment difference represents a change from a 50% to a 63% 5-year disease-free survival rate; not an unimportant difference. Thus, between 200 and 300 patients are required per treatment program to provide definitive results. At times, independent treatment comparisons within biologically distinct patient subgroups (e.g., based on menopausal status) are desired. In this situation, a large number of patients must be entered from each subgroup of interest. Adjuvant programs are often applied to patient populations which have a relatively long disease-free survival even without the addition of chemotherapy. Therefore, a long period of follow-up of all patients is required to determine the ultimate impact of the adjuvant chemotherapy.

Principal Differences Between Conventional Adjuvant Trials and Perioperative Trials

The major difference between conventional adjuvant chemotherapy trials and perioperative chemotherapy trials is the crucial role of timing of drug administration. Figure 1 shows the schema for a conventional adjuvant trial. Adjuvant chemotherapy is to start within 6 weeks after surgery. There is time to carry out several critical activities before the patient is actually entered into the study at randomization. Postoperative patient recovery, pathology information, special laboratory studies, eligibility confirmation, patient consent, stratification data, and consultation with a medical oncologist can all be obtained during this period. The status of the patient and that of the disease are well established by the time the patient enters the trial. The comparison of Regimen A with Regimen B will be carried out for those patients who reach the point of randomization and enter the study as shown in Fig. 1.

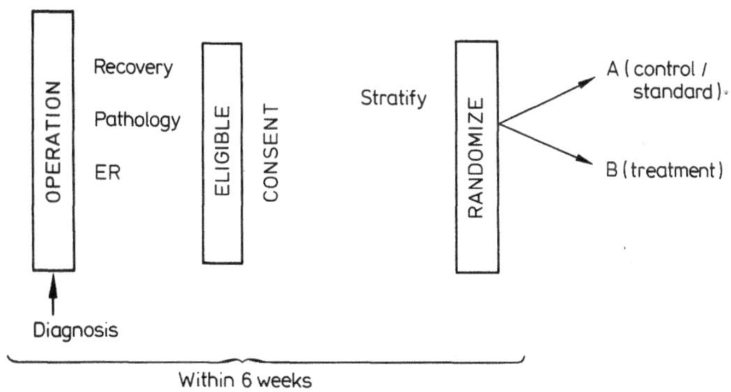

Fig. 1. Design for trials of conventionally timed adjuvant chemotherapy

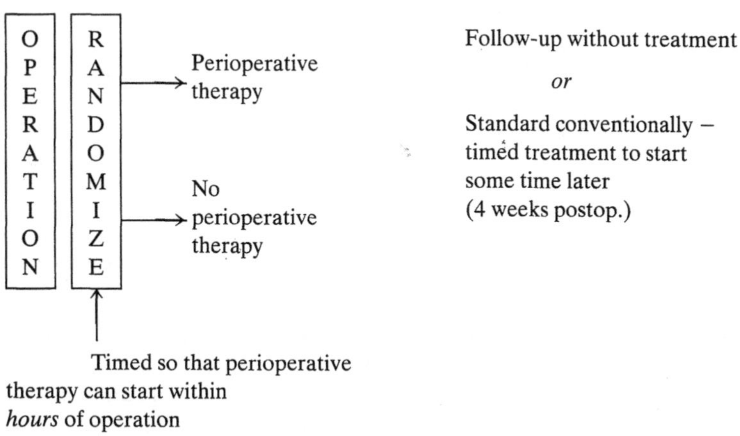

Fig. 2. Design for trial of perioperative adjuvant chemotherapy

In contrast, Fig. 2 shows the schema for a trial designed to evaluate the effectiveness of perioperative chemotherapy. In this case, the randomization must be performed and the patient must enter the trial so that the perioperative therapy can start within *hours* rather than within weeks of the operation. The requirement for initiation of adjuvant therapy soon after operation presents several logistic difficulties setting these trials apart from conventional adjuvant trials, some of which are listed below.

1. The mechanism of patient entry must avoid delays in treatment assignment.
2. Patient eligibility may not be completely established at the time of study entry.
3. The design may require a forced delay of chemotherapy for some patients.
4. Important prognostic factors that might influence the choice of treatment may not be known prior to randomization.
5. The patient population entering a perioperative trial will be different from the usual adjuvant population, yielding biased comparisons with published results of adjuvant chemotherapy trials.

The currently active trial of the Ludwig Breast Cancer Study Group (1981) can be used as an example to illustrate the issues listed above. The Ludwig Breast Cancer Study Group is an international cooperative group with participating clinics in Australia, Germany, New Zealand, South Africa, Spain, Sweden, Switzerland, and Yugoslavia. The coordinating center is in Bern, Switzerland, and the statistical center is in Amherst, NY, USA and Boston, Mass, USA. In October 1981, the Group completed entry of over 1700 patients with operable breast cancer into four clinical trials (studies I–IV) designed to evaluate chemotherapy and hormonotherapy as adjuvant treatments. Patients have been entering the current trial (study V) since November 1981. The study design for the project (Perioperative and Conventionally Timed Chemotherapy in Operable Breast Cancer) is shown in Fig. 3. The key features are (a) that randomization must occur so that perioperative chemotherapy can begin within 36 hours of completion of the operation; and (b) the nodal status of the patient will not be known prior to the commencement of perioperative therapy and will influence the type of subsequent treatment delivered.

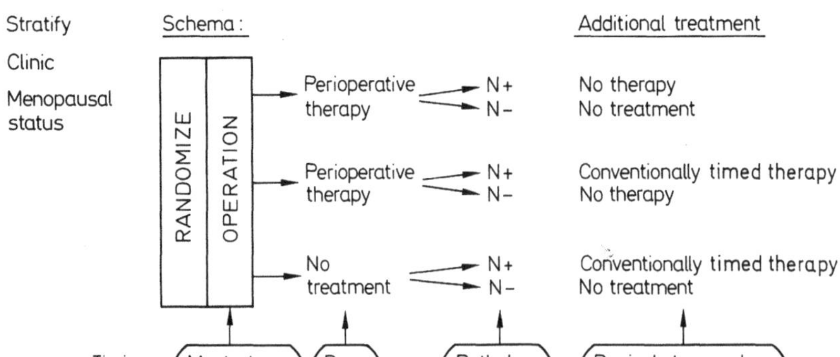

Fig. 3. Design of Ludwig Breast Cancer Study Group's Study V: Perioperative and conventionally timed chemotherapy in operable breast cancer. Perioperative therapy, CMF by IV route, started within 36 hours of completion of the operation, plus leucovorin; conventionally timed therapy. CMFp with TAM for 6 months in postmenopausal patients and CMFp alone for 6 months in premenopausal patients, starting not less than 25 days after surgery

Logistics of Patient Entry

To allow perioperative treatment to be given within 36 hours of mastectomy, it is necessary to have a satisfactory system for rapid central registration and randomization. The possible mechanisms for randomization into the trial are illustrated in Fig. 4. The three alternative approaches are

1. Randomization carried out *prior to mastectomy* but after a histologically *confirmed diagnosis* of breast cancer obtained either by open biopsy or by needle biopsy.
2. Randomization carried out immediately *after mastectomy* so that chemotherapy can be given on the first postoperative day.
3. Randomization carried out prior to mastectomy and *before* a *histological diagnosis* has been obtained. If the patient's breast lesion is found to be benign, then trial entry is cancelled by submitting Form A–X with the clinic's pathology report to the Operations Office.

The above three mechanisms for randomization were established so that all clinics could participate in the perioperative trial regardless of institutional policies concerning the management of these patients.
In Ludwig Breast Cancer Study Group studies I–IV, treatment assignments were obtained by telephone or telex to the Central Operations Office in Bern. The group felt that central randomization, which provides for controlled study entry and efficient data flow scheduling, was an important feature of a cooperative group effort (Stanley et al. 1981). Because of the necessity for rapid treatment assignment in study V, some investigators argued that the sealed envelope system maintained at each individual institution for randomization could be used. The group, however, decided that central control of registration and randomization was important to maintain the quality and credibility of the study. To avoid the time delays involved in such a global trial, a second centralized randomization unit was established in Sydney for patient entries from Australia and New Zealand. As the randomization is stratified by menopausal status and institution, having a separate center for a group of institutions presents no problems.

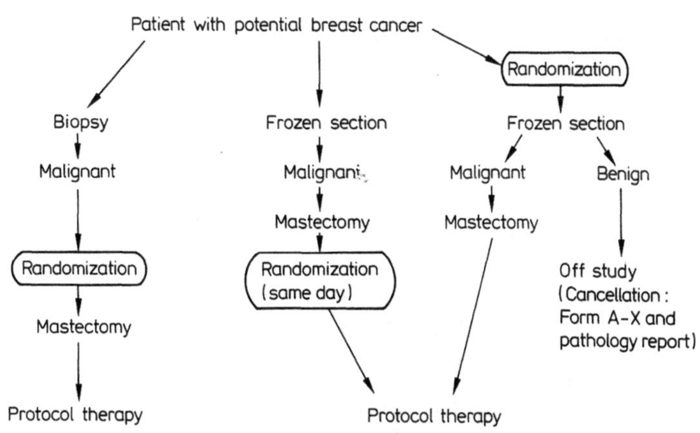

Fig. 4. Timing of randomization to allow initiation of perioperative therapy within 36 hours of mastectomy

Unknown Patient Eligibility at the Time of Study Entry

One of the three mechanisms for patient entry outlined above involves the randomization of patients prior to histological diagnosis of malignancy. A patient subsequently found to have benign disease is removed from the study as a so-called A–X cancellation. To avoid the possibility of unbalanced numbers of ineligible patients entering the different treatment arms, it was suggested that the treatments for cancelled cases be reassigned to future study entries. While this practice would avoid imbalances, there are several difficulties with its implementation. The reassignment of treatments may introduce additional complexities and opportunities for errors in the randomization process. Furthermore, there is a time delay in the appropriate review of A–X cases. Finally, in a large trial with a low A–X rate such a balancing procedure is unnecessary. For example, if 50 patients were entered per treatment and the A–X rate were 20%, imbalances more extreme than 47, 40, and 33 eligible patients per arm would occur less than 1% of the time. As over 500 entries per treatment are planned for study V, and an A–X rate well below 20% is anticipated, reassignment of A–X cancellation treatments appears to be unnecessary.
The status of the randomization scheme as of 30 September 1982 is shown in Table 1. Less than 5% of the randomizations have been cancelled as A–X patients. Of the patients admitted so far, 33% were randomized before the mastectomy, 44% were randomized on the day of the mastectomy, and 18% were randomized on the day after the mastectomy. Almost 20% of the patients entered the trial prior to histological confirmation of breast cancer.

Required Delay of Chemotherapy

Another potential difficulty with the perioperative trial is the fact that patients who do not receive perioperative therapy are required to have their conventionally timed adjuvant therapy some time later. Dose 1 of perioperative treatment must begin within *36 hours* after mastectomy, while other patients are to receive the first dose of conventionally timed treatment no sooner than *25 days* after mastectomy. If these timing requirements are violated to any substantial degree the impact of the perioperative and conventionally timed

Table 1. Registration status of Ludwig Breast Cancer Study Group's study V as of 30 September 1982

581	Entries (15 Nov. 81 to 30 Sept. 82)
43	Awaiting data
538	
26	A–X Cancellations (< 5%)
180	Randomized before mastectomy (39 without histological confirmation)
234	Randomized on same day (37 without histological confirmation)
98	Randomized on next day

adjuvants will begin to blend together. Thus, control over the timing of therapy in addition to the other aspects of treatment administration is crucial for adequate evaluation of therapeutic differences.

Important Prognostic Features May not Be Known Prior to Randomization

Because randomization must occur prior to the availability of the results of complete pathology and other laboratory studies (ER status), many important prognostic features of the patient will not be known prior to randomization. Therefore, these factors cannot be used to stratify the randomization. The lack of this information at randomization may influence design considerations that relate to subsequent treatment. For study V, whether a patient has positive or negative axillary node involvement is unknown at the time of randomization. Under the current design shown in Fig. 3, on average two-thirds of the node-negative patients will receive perioperative chemotherapy. Some investigators felt that this might represent "over-treating" a majority of the node-negative patients. It was suggested that the study design might be revised so that only one-half of the patients would be assigned to perioperative chemotherapy. This revised design would involve a second randomization for patients who were subsequently found to have positive axillary node involvement. The percentages of the population allocated to each treatment for the current design and the revised design are shown in Table 2. While the revised design is preferred for the node-negative patients, inefficiencies are introduced for the treatment evaluation among node-positive patients. Because only half of the patients are assigned to perioperative treatment, the comparison of perioperative treatment only versus perioperative plus conventionally timed adjuvant treatment is conducted at reduced efficiency. One-third more node-positive patients would have to enter the trial to provide the same strength for the comparison as in the original design. In addition, the logistic complexities of conducting a second randomization are prohibitive. Thus, the current design is used, in which two-thirds of all patients receive perioperative chemotherapy.

Table 2. Comparison of current design and suggested revision of study V

		Percentage of population	
		Current design	*Revised design*
N^+	Perioperative chemotherapy alone	33%	25%
	Perioperative + conventionally timed chemotherapy	33%	25%
	Conventionally timed chemotherapy alone	33%	50%
N^-	Perioperative chemotherapy alone	67%	50%
	No adjuvant treatment	33%	50%

Revised design *balances N^- study and improves efficiency*
(requires 0.89 of original sample size)
but, comparison of *perioperative chemotherapy alone versus perioperative + conventionally timed chemotherapy has reduced efficiency*
(requires 1.33 of original sample size)

Difference Between Patient Populations in Perioperative Chemotherapy Trials and in Conventional Adjuvant Chemotherapy Trials

Because patient entry occurs earlier in perioperative chemotherapy trials than in conventional adjuvant studies, the patient populations may be different. Figure 5 illustrates various ways in which patients who enter perioperative studies might have been excluded from entry into a conventional adjuvant trial. Patients with surgical morbidity or mortality enter the perioperative program but would not enter the standard adjuvant study. Similarly, laboratory and pathology findings, additional work-up procedures, and the opportunity for patients to withdraw consent prior to randomization may affect the entry of patients into an adjuvant program. Thus, the results of perioperative trials should not be compared with the published results of other adjuvant studies.
It is particularly important to avoid comparison of postoperative complications between patients who receive perioperative chemotherapy and patients who receive standard adjuvant therapy. Wound healing problems may exclude patients from receiving conventional adjuvant therapy. On the other hand, wound healing problems might be observed more often with perioperative treatment just because the patients are being observed more frequently and more carefully. Comparisons on the impact of treatment must be made in comparable patient groups that are subject to comparable follow-up schedules and evaluations.

Analysis by "Intent to Treat" Is Required to Yield Unbiased Results

Many things that are beyond the control of the investigator can happen after the randomized allocation of treatment. Patients may withdraw their consent to receive treatment, surgical morbidity or mortality may prevent the patient from receiving the assigned treatment, or various errors in treatment administration may occur. Because these patients did not receive the assigned treatment program, an investigator may feel justified in excluding them from the analysis of results. Figure 6 illustrates the situation in which

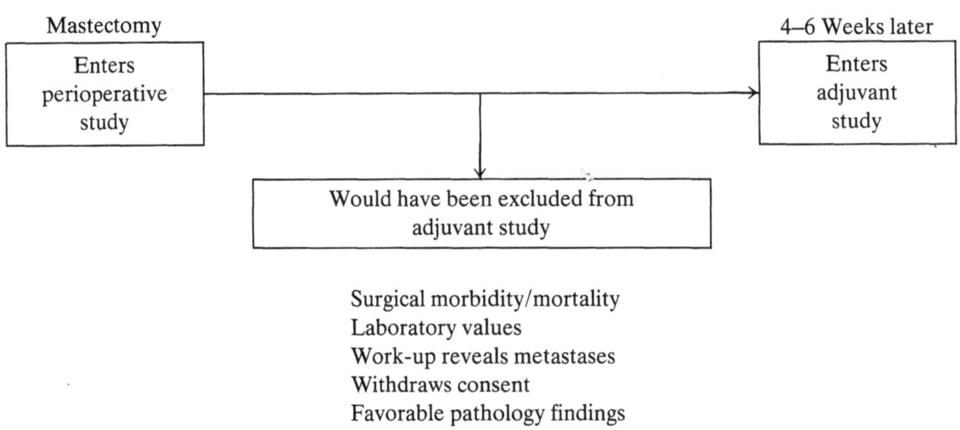

Fig. 5. Reasons why results of perioperative adjuvant chemotherapy trials should not be compared with published results of studies of other adjuvant therapies

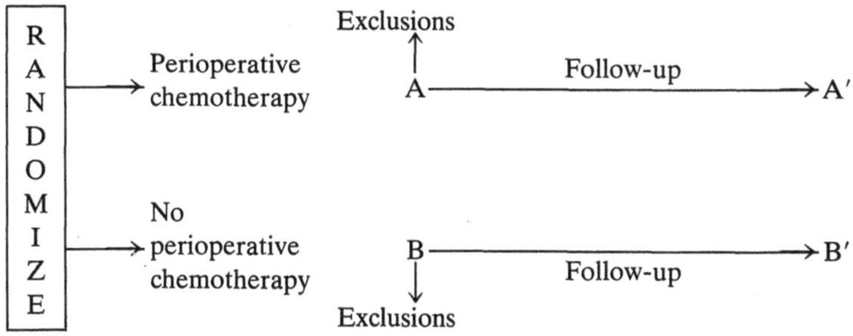

Fig. 6. Case exclusions and follow-up. Groups A and B, established by randomization, are alike on average, so that any differences observed are treatment effects. But A' and B' may not be similarly comparable. Analysis by intent to treat is needed for an unbiased comparison of treatment programs

patients have been excluded from consideration prior to data analysis. Treatment groups A and B are assumed following randomization to be "alike on average" in all aspects that are likely to influence the results. In this way, observed differences between the outcome for group A versus group B are likely to represent real treatment differences. If, however, patients are excluded from the analysis for various reasons which may be treatment related, then groups A' and B' may not be comparable in this way. Selection biases, which were controlled by the randomization, may be introduced by the subsequent exclusion of patients. For example, the comparison of perioperative treatment alone with conventionally timed adjuvant therapy may be biased if patients who fail to receive the perioperative treatment within 36 hours of mastectomy are excluded from the analysis. These patients may represent a poor prognostic group if late starting has been due to concurrent medical problems. The concept of analysis by intent to treat has therefore been recommended as a way of avoiding the potential biases introduced by case exclusions (Peto et al. 1977). In an intent-to-treat analysis, all patients are evaluated as members of the randomized treatment group regardless of the treatment actually received. The results of such an analysis reflect the impact of the recommendation for one treatment program versus the other treatment program. This is the comparison for which the randomized trial was designed, as a management study rather than as an explanatory study (Sackett and Gent 1979). If a large fraction of the patients are excluded owing to failure to receive the assigned treatment, this in itself will provide information about the treatment's feasibility. However, to exclude these patients and then compare the remaining cases with those who have received the other treatment regimen may clearly yield a biased comparison for the application of the treatment in the overall population.

The intent-to-treat analysis is particularly important for trials of perioperative chemotherapy. Because patients enter these trials around the time of surgery there are many opportunities for patients to fail to receive the precise treatment. Surgical morbidity and mortality may interfere with treatment administration. Unavoidable delays may prevent the timely administration of the perioperative treatment. The availability of subsequent additional information from the pathology department and other sources may alter the willingness of the physician or the patient to continue with the assigned therapy program. Because of these and other factors, analysis by intent to treat is required for unbiased results to be obtained in perioperative chemotherapy trials. *All patients are to be followed up and accounted for in the analysis, regardless of treatment actually received.* No cancellations (with the exception of documented A–X patients) are allowed. The conclusions from such an analysis are representative of a recommended treatment policy. The ability to carry out the assigned treatment program represents another facet of the analysis.

Conclusion

This paper has discussed some of the methodological issues relating to the conduct of perioperative chemotherapy trials and highlighted some of the similarities between perioperative trials and the usual adjuvant situations. These include the requirement for sound study design, including randomization as the mechanism for assigning treatment to patients. Large numbers of patients followed for prolonged periods of time are also required. In addition to these basic concepts, perioperative chemotherapy trials involve special logistic difficulties related to the requirements imposed by the timing of treatment administration. Key data items will be unknown at the time of randomization. Populations of patients who enter perioperative chemotherapy trials will differ from those who enter conventional adjuvant programs. Finally, the importance of an analysis by intent to treat is particularly relevant for perioperative chemotherapy trials. Only by such an analysis can we appreciate the true impact of the perioperative treatment program in practice.

Summary

Cancer clinical trials designed to test the value of perioperative chemotherapy present special statistical problems for the investigator. Because chemotherapy must begin within hours of surgery, aspects of the design, conduct, and analysis of such trials are more complex than for many other types of clinical investigations. Special attention must be given to the logistics of patient entry. In some situations, patients may receive a treatment assignment prior to the determination of eligibility or even prior to histological diagnosis of cancer. Design problems may arise when important prognostic factors are not known at the time of randomization. A comparison of perioperative chemotherapy to other, conventionally timed adjuvant chemotherapy requires that adjuvant treatment be purposely delayed for some patients. Because patients enter a perioperative chemotherapy trial before or soon after surgery, the patient population is not the same as that treated in standard adjuvant trials. Thus it is not possible to compare results directly between perioperative and standard adjuvant trials. Analyses of toxicity will include surgical morbidity which would not be seen in conventional adjuvant trials. The analysis of perioperative chemotherapy trials requires care, as many case exclusion factors may make it difficult to determine the true effectiveness of the perioperative treatment plan. Analysis by intent to treat is recommended. These and other statistical and logistic aspects are discussed with reference to the current trial being conducted by the Ludwig Breast Cancer Study Group.

References

Byar DP (1979) The necessity and justification of randomized clinical trials. In: Tagnon HJ, Staquet MD (eds) Controversies in cancer – design of trials and treatment. Masson, New York

Chalmers TC, Block JB, Lee S (1972) Controlled studies in clinical cancer research. N Engl J Med 297: 1091–1096

Freiman JA, Chalmers TC, Smith H, Kuebler RR (1978) The importance of beta, the type II error and sample size in the design and interpretation of the randomized control trial. N Engl J Med 299: 690–694

Ludwig Breast Cancer Study Group (1981) Study V: protocol for perioperative and conventionally-timed chemotherapy in operable breast cancer. Activated: 13 november 1981; revised: may and november 1982. Ludwig Institute for Cancer Research, Bern

Peto R, Pike MC, Armitage P, Breslow NE, Cox DR, Howard SV, Mantel N, McPherson K, Peto J, Smith PG (1976) Design and analysis of randomized clinical trials requiring prolonged observation of each patient. I. Introduction and design. Br J Cancer 34: 585–612

Peto R, Pike MC, Armitage P, Breslow NE, Cox DR, Howard SV, Mantel N, McPherson K, Peto J, Smith PG (1977) Design and analysis of randomized clinical trials requiring prolonged observation of each patient. II. Analysis and examples. Br J Cancer 35: 1–39

Sackett DL, Gent M (1979) Controversy in counting and attributing events in clinical trials. N Engl J Med 301: 1410–1414

Stanley K, Stjernsward J, Isley M (1981) The conduct of a cooperative clinical trial. Springer Berlin Heidelberg New York. (recent results in cancer research, vol 77)

Zelen M (1983) Guidelines for publishing papers on cancer clinical trials: responsibilities of editors and authors. J Clin Oncol 1: 164–169

What Is Perioperative Chemotherapy?

The first panel discussion at the Symposium dealt with the definition of perioperative chemotherapy and with the aims of this combined-modality approach to cancer. Perioperative chemotherapy – in a broad sense – includes any chemotherapy around the time of surgery, e.g., preoperative, intraoperative, and immediately postoperative chemotherapy. Most surgeons would agree that perioperative measures, by definition, are those that interfere with the surgical procedure itself by influencing surgical morbidity through clotting activity, immunocompetence, wound healing, etc. Depending on the chemotherapy regimen used and the surgery performed, this perioperative period may be only 1 or 2 days in one case, or a few weeks or even months in other instances. Therefore, it was unanimously felt that this type of functional definition of perioperative chemotherapy is not suitable for oncologic practice. At this point, some participants proposed omission of the term perioperative and a clear statement of the timing of chemotherapy as preoperative, intraoperative, or immediate postoperative. Based on the rationale of perioperative chemotherapy (see below) given as an *adjuvant* to potentially curative surgery, it was concluded that, more strictly speaking, perioperative chemotherapy should be started as soon as possible *after* tumor resection. Usually, surgery is the best tool in establishing the histopathological diagnosis, in staging the extent of disease, and in reducing the tumor mass to a minimal tumor burden. Furthermore, chemotherapy given before surgery may lead to an unnecessary delay of potentially curative resection at least in nonresponding patients. Based on the *purposes* of perioperative chemotherapy – curative tumor cell kill by the best available chemotherapy with the lowest total body burden of tumor stem cells – chemotherapy should be started as soon as possible, preferably at the time of surgery.

Preoperative Chemotherapy: Advantages and Clinical Application in Stage III Breast Cancer*

A. N. Papaioannou**

The Mount Vernon Hospital, 12 North Seventh Avenue, Mont Vernon, NY 10550, USA

Introduction

The inability to control the micrometastases present at the diagnosis of breast cancer (BC) accounts for most if not all of our present treatment failures. Even if only patients with localized breast cancer are considered, up to 40% will die of their tumor within 10 years (Nealon et al. 1979). The survival rate even for patients with the most favorable prognosis (with negative nodes) at 40 years is 53%, whereas the corresponding figure for those with positive nodes is 19% (Rutqvist and Wallgren 1982). In fact if all patients who develop breast cancer are followed until death, systemic breast cancer may be found to be the ultimate cause of death in as many as 90% of them (Mueller et al. 1978; Langlands et al. 1979; Henderson and Canellos 1980). In stage III (locally advanced) BC, from a practical standpoint all patients harbor micrometastases, and as a rule the end-result is death due to this disease (Papaioannou and Urban 1964; Pearlman et al. 1976; Osteen et al. 1978; Terz et al. 1978). Attempts to achieve more effective control of the latent systemic spread of BC are currently being made in many clinical trials based on various adjuvant regimens with cytostatic and/or hormonal agents. In practically all studies in which chemotherapy is used, treatment begins a few weeks after the operation. This policy of delaying treatment of the systemic component of the disease until after operation may be disadvantageous however. A good reason for suspecting this is supplied by observations showing that in an experimental setting micrometastases begin to grow faster immediately after the primary focus is eliminated. This change in tumor behavior has been observed repeatedly in a variety of tumor models since the beginning of the century (Tyzzer 1913), both after surgical removal of the primary tumor (Tyzzer 1913; Schatton 1958; Ketcham et al. 1959, 1961; DeWys 1972; Simpson-Herren et al. 1976; Gorelik et al. 1978; Gunduz et al. 1979) and after its destruction by irradiation (Kaplan and Murphy 1948; Van den Brenk and Sharpington 1971; Sheldon and Fowler 1973). In the experimental animal this kinetic change apparently occurs within 24 hours and is no longer evident 7 days later (Gunduz et al. 1979). To our knowledge, similar clinical observations have been made repeatedly in

* Supported by Contract No. 79021 from the Service of Scientific Research and Development of the Ministry of Coordination and by funds from the Hellenic Cancer Society

** For the Hellenic Breast Cooperative Group; the members of the Group are listed in Appendix 1. AP's present address is Department of Surgery, Mt. Vernon Hospital, Mt. Vernon, NY 10550, USA

Recent Results in Cancer Research. Vol. 98

oncologic practice, although anecdotally. At any rate, since this phenomenon has been reported in a substantial number of experimental systems it should arouse concern as to its possible occurrence also in man. Particularly after resection of primary BC, if micrometastases are present as often as the evidence suggests, and are indeed enhanced immediately after operation, the consequences could be grave.

The exact mechanism of this micrometastatic enhancement in the immediate postoperative period is uncertain, but there are various possibilities. It may, for example, be a manifestation of a tumor cell-to-cell interaction between the heterogeneous subpopulations of the same tumor, as some studies suggest (DeWys 1972; Simpson-Herren et al. 1976; Gorelik et al. 1978). The mechanism of this interaction is probably immunological in nature (Miller et al. 1980). The soluble growth factors secreted and utilized by tumors (Sporr and Todaro 1980; Sherwin et al. 1981) may also be responsible to some extent for the interactions between tumor cell subpopulations. Other studies have documented a number of tumor-enhancing factors at work during the perioperative period, which may strengthen existing micrometastases and facilitate the development of new ones. Immunosuppression due to surgical injury and anesthetic and other drugs used before or after operation, for example, can all reduce cell-mediated immunity (CMI) and experimentally increase the metastatic potential of the tumor (Papaioannou 1981c). Likewise, immunosuppressive peptides, which appear in the circulation shortly after major operations (McLaughlin et al. 1979), may accelerate tumor growth. Reduction of the reticuloendothelial system function and hypoopsonemia also lead to further depression of CMI after major operations and experimentally favor tumor growth (Saba 1978). In addition, perioperative changes in the coagulability of the blood may favor the development of new micrometastases (Zacharski et al. 1979). Even the perioperative anxiety and postoperative depression associated with mastectomy, not unlike other stresses of modern life inducing immune suppression (Ader 1980), may influence the tumor-host relationship in the same direction. Experimentally, emotional, psychosocial, or anxiety-stimulated stress produces neuroendocrine changes affecting the immunological apparatus and ultimately the host resistance to cancer (Riley 1981; Newberry 1981). Some of these emotional factors may also be operative in man in many subtile ways, and every effort should be made to prevent them as far as possible (Papaioannou 1982).

From these introductory thoughts we can conclude, then, that if the microscopic metastatic foci of BC are indeed entrenched perioperatively it would be reasonable to shift our *initial* therapeutic attention from the primary site of BC to its systemic component. In support of this notion, we discuss below the theoretical advantages of treating the systemic component of BC as soon as the diagnosis is made and present supporting experimental and clinical evidence, including our own studies indicating that systemic treatment used before operation is safe in a variety of operable solid tumors in man; indeed it may be more effective than the reverse treatment sequence now practiced. Finally we will review our results with a more recent prospective study evaluating chemoendocrine systemic therapy used before mastectomy with or without postoperative radiotherapy in locally advanced (stage III) BC.

Conceptual Advantages of Preoperative Chemotherapy

A number of theoretical considerations can be adduced to support the view that preoperative chemotherapy (Preop. ch.) is more beneficial than the postoperative adjuvant chemotherapy now under study in a great variety of schemes throughout the world.

Interference with the Potential for Metastasis

Cell variants destined to form metastases pre-exist in the primary tumor (Fidler and Kripke 1977). If these cells are left with intact potential and are forced into the circulation at operation they are likely to establish new micrometastases in a distal organ or locally, particularly under the conditions of perioperative hypercoagulability and immunosuppression mentioned above. Chemotherapy, however, will primarily affect actively growing cells, so that a 50% reduction in the size of the primary tumor will decrease clonogenic cells by more than 99.9% (Fisher 1977). It follows, then, that if surgery is carried out after systemic chemotherapy has practically eliminated clonogenic cells, the primary tumor will be lacking in cells with the potential to form metastases. Once effective systemic therapy is given, preoperative and intraoperative cancer cell dissemination will become an inconsequential event.

Provision of a Tumor Chemosensitivity Test In Vivo

Our present inability to test tumor chemosensitivity with accuracy in vitro, despite all current efforts (Selby et al. 1983; von Hoff 1983), is entirely understandable in view of the cellular heterogeneity of tumors and the extreme complexity of the in vivo events leading to remission. Conversely, observation of the primary tumor after systemic therapy is given will in effect be measuring the end-result of the interaction between all pharmacological, neoplastic, and host factors involved in the process of remission. Thus preoperative chemotherapy could be used as a very simple, fast, inexpensive and, hopefully, effective means of estimating chemosensitivity in vivo. An additional advantage would be that a possible chemosensitivity would be known from the very start of therapy and not, as now happens with postoperative adjuvant therapy, when the disease ultimately recurs.

Prevention of Development of Drug-Resistant Clones

The probability of cure by chemotherapy diminishes and is ultimately lost as tumor burden increases (Burchenal 1976). This may be related, among other things, to the spontaneous development of drug-resistant clones, the absolute numbers and proportions of which will increase with time. It has been estimated that the likelihood that at least one chemotherapy-resistant cell will develop increases sharply over a short interval during the early phases of tumor growth (Goldie and Coldman 1979). It has been also shown experimentally (Skipper et al. 1964) that the composition of micrometastases can change, over several volume-doubling times, from containing predominantly drug-sensitive cells to mainly drug-resistant cells. These drug-resistant mutations may ultimately prove to be as important in the chemotherapy of tumors as they are in the management of microbial infections.

Prevention of Escape Mechanisms from Immune Tumor Destruction

Early systemic therapy may also assist the host to suppress mechanisms of tumor escape from immune destruction, which facilitate metastases and favor local growth. Many such mechanisms depend on tumor-elaborated substances, e.g., antigenic determinants shed from the tumor cell surface (Currie and Alexander 1974), the tumor angiogenesis factor, inducing the development of tumor microcirculation (Folkman and Cotran 1976), and substances suppressing macrophage function (Pike and Snyderman 1976) or inhibiting macrophage chemotaxis (North et al. 1976). Since all these substances are products of active cells, and chemotherapy has adverse effects on cellular functions, it is reasonable to assume that cytotoxic chemotherapy could inhibit their production. Suppressor cells may also contribute to tumor growth (Broder and Waldman 1978). Some of these cells, however, and particularly T cell suppressors, are sensitive to chemotherapy, and it is on this basis that under certain conditions such treatment may stimulate immune responses rather than the reverse (Rollinghoff et al. 1977). The growth of small metastatic clusters may therefore be enhanced during the perioperative period, but arrested or subdued through perioperative chemotherapy, by inhibiting any or all of these tumor-enhancing mechanisms.

Prevention of Increase in Tumor Burden

The currently usual interval of about 1 month from diagnosis to the beginning of postoperative systemic treatment may allow an increase of about 30% in the microscopic tumor burden, assuming an average doubling time for breast cancer of 90 days at the time of diagnosis (Steel 1977).

This estimate, however, may be conservative in view of the likelihood that micrometastases may grow faster than their respective primaries and that the immunosuppressive effect of operation, emotional stress, drugs, and possibly the other factors at work perioperatively, as discussed above, may accelerate the growth of microscopic deposits. The above delay in initiation of systemic treatment is therefore likely to be far more detrimental to patients harboring anaplastic tumors with shorter doubling times and greater metastatic potential than to those with slow-growing neoplasms which tend to remain localized. The exact percentage of fast-growing tumors (defined as those detected within 13 months after a negative examination) is not known. However, in a recent estimate of breast cancers found from serial mammograms in a screening population of 10,120 women, as many as 77% of women affected may fall in this subset with fast-growing tumors; these have twice as high an incidence of positive nodes at surgery as their counterparts with slow-growing tumors (Heuser et al. 1979).

Exploitation of Prerequisites for Maximum Tumor Chemosensitivity

A number of other kinetic considerations favor the notion that systemic treatment at the earliest possible time increases the likelihood of eliminating disseminated disease. The microscopic metastatic foci, for example, have their smallest possible volume in each patient at the time the diagnosis is made. The smaller they are, the greater the likelihood that they will divide more actively, have a larger surface area in relation to their volume, a more homogeneous cell population, and a rich oxygen supply, and not have a reduced level of accumulated metabolites capable of inhibiting the effects of chemotherapeutic agents (Frei 1977). At this stage, therefore, microscopic foci are presumably easily synchronizable and more vulnerable to cell-cycle-specific drugs (Schabel 1977). Likewise, according to the Norton-Simon hypothesis (1977), the chemosensitivity of tumors is greatest at the inflection point of the Gomperzian growth curve of tumors. This point is found just before or at the time the clinical diagnosis is made. Maximum tumor chemosensitivity can also be achieved if chemotherapy is used before operation, because of the intact vascularity of the tumor and consequently better drug delivery. At this time the better general condition of the host in terms of physical, nutritional and emotional status, leading to better drug tolerance, is also likely to enhance the overall responce to chemotherapy.

Suitability for Use as an Immunostimulating Agent

The immunosuppressive effects of cytotoxic agents do not preclude their use before operation. In fact, if used preoperatively they have a theoretical advantage that may increase their value as therapeutic agents. After completion of a short intensive chemotherapy course immunity is depressed, but it gradually recovers in the 2nd week and ultimately "rebounds" to levels higher than the pretreatment levels of function, where it is maintained for another week (Harris et al. 1976).

If the operation is timed to take place during this last phase of heightened immunity, preoperative chemotherapy can be exploited as a systemic immunostimulating agent. This in turn may offset, at least in part, the suppressive effects of surgery on immunity and reticuloendothelial system function.

Possible Elimination or Limitation of Need for Mastectomy or Irradiation

It is easy to see how primary tumors successfully treated initially by chemotherapy are reduced in size, have a considerably lower blood supply, and consequently may require less extensive surgery for eradication. Partial mastectomy with or without axillary lymphadenectomy or simple tumorectomy may be entirely adequate for that purpose. In these circumstances, local irradiation may replace resection. In fact, if more effective cytostatic agents are discovered the need for resection or irradiation may be entirely eliminated. Evidence that these possibilities may be real is provided by the ability to salvage sarcoma-bearing limbs, which previously had to be amputated (Morton et al. 1976; Rosen et al. 1978), or perform less extensive surgery or radiotherapy following initial chemotherapy in a variety of head and neck cancers (Tarpley et al. 1975; Frei 1982). On the basis of the considerations discussed above, at best the subclinical component of solid tumors would be totally eliminated after preoperative chemotherapy and the primary deprived of cells with the potential to metastasize. Thus the possibility of cure will increase markedly. At worst, the growth of existing and new micrometastases would be curtailed to a limited degree only, and postoperative adjuvant chemotherapy would be imperative. Even in this case, however, subsequent treatment would be directed against a smaller overall microscopic tumor burden than that logically expected to be present if adjuvant therapy is delayed for a few weeks after operation. At any rate, the combination of preoperative and postoperative chemotherapy is more likely than the latter alone to reduce the overall micrometastatic mass below the critical volume which is necessary for tumor regrowth (Fig. 1). Immune mechanisms, either alone or aided by stimulating agents after operation, can be more efficient in eradicating any remaining subclinical disease or holding it in check when it is truly minimal.

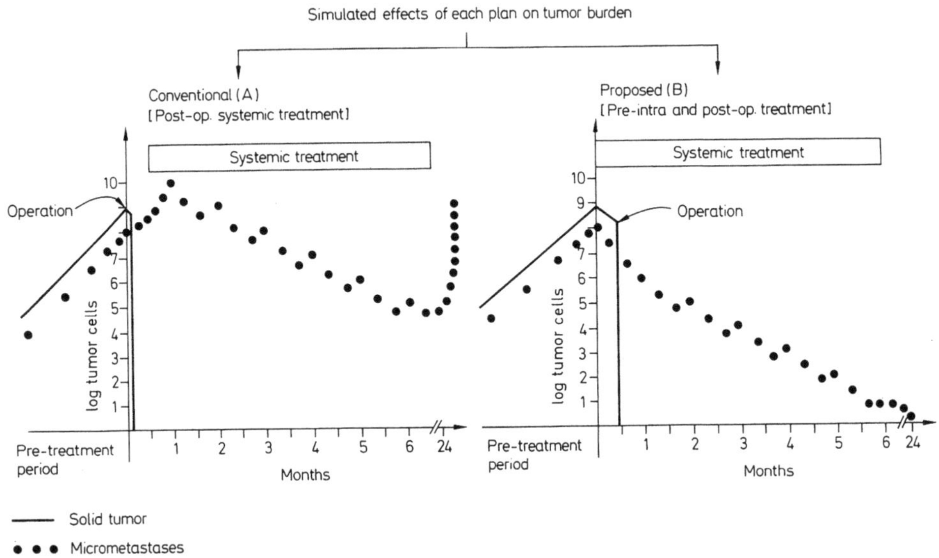

Fig. 1. Comparison of conventional and proposed treatments. All effects of both therapeutic plans depicted are hypothetical. Exponential growth is assumed for both the primary tumor and its micrometastases before diagnosis is made. In the absence of chemotherapy, enhancement of micrometastases in the immediate postoperative period is evident in the conventional plan (*A*). (See *Introduction* and section: *Prevention of Increase in Tumor Burden.*) In the proposed plan (*B*) one log reduction of tumor cells corresponds to about 50% reduction in size of the primary tumor. Since this reduction in size is primarily achieved by destruction of actively dividing cells, in a tumor shrinking by 50% practically all clonogenic cells are eliminated *(Interference with the Potential for Metastasis).* In plan B operation is timed to take place during the rebound of immunity that follows the initial phase of postchemotherapy immunosuppression *(Suitability for use as Immunostimulating Agent).* Postoperative chemotherapy begins against a much smaller micrometastatic load in plan *B* than in plan *A*. Ultimate cytoreduction in plan *B* is below the presumed critical volume necessary for tumor regrowth. At this point immune mechanisms hold in check on extirpate remaining microscopic foci, effecting clinical cure. In plan *A* this critical level of cytoreduction may not be achieved and micrometastases are more likely to grow unrestrained and kill the host (Papaioannou 1981a)

Factual Evidence

A variety of experimental and clinical studies have documented the value of preoperative chemotherapy in the treatment of solid tumors in general and of breast cancer in particular. These data were found to be scattered in the literature over more than two decades. Some of this evidence has been previously reviewed (Papaioannou 1981b) and is presented here in greater detail.

Experimental Data

Twenty-five years ago Brock (1959) used the transplantable Shay chloroleukoma of the rat, a widely metastasizing tumor, which is 100% lethal if left without treatment. Surgical excision of the tumor is associated with a 23% cure rate. If the animals are treated with 30 mg/kg cyclophosphamide IV twice the cure rate is 28%. When the first cyclophosphamide injection is given 1 hour before operation and the second 24 hours after operation, 50% of the animals survive. If the above two doses of cyclophosphamide are given 8 and 7 days before tumor excision 90% of these animals are cured (Brock 1959). To our knowledge this was the first experimental evidence of benefit derived by preoperative chemotherapy, documented 25 years ago. Almost 10 years later, Karrer et al. (1967), using the Lewis lung tumor in BDF1 mice in a variety of preoperative and postoperative combinations of adjuvant treatment schedules, showed a linear dose-response curve when chemotherapy was begun 2 days before amputation of the tumor-bearing extremity and was continued for 5 days thereafter. When 30 mg/kg cyclophosphamide was given, 100% of the animals survived; when the dose was progressively lowered survival proportionately decreased. Subsequently Bogden et al. (1974), using a spontaneously metastasizing adenocarcinoma in Fisher rats, which is 100% lethal when treated by surgical excision only, showed that chemotherapy given on the day of surgery or 10 days before surgery cured 70%–80% of the animals. Likewise, Pendergrast et al. (1976), using multiple experiments in the B16 melanoma in C57BL mice, showed that the combination of a single course of chemotherapy preceding surgery increased survival from 38%–43% in controls to 50.5%–87.9% in treated animals. Two other, more recent, studies are also noteworthy. In a mouse model with simulated metastases, Fisher et al. (1979) observed an advantage in treating the "metastatic" disease first by various chemoimmunotherapy regimens and delaying removal of the primary tumor. Likewise, Schabel et al. (1979a) recorded 63% cures of a transplanted metastasizing murine tumor when adriamycin was given 12 days after implantation and resection was performed on day 15. However, if adriamycin was given on day 18 (3 days postoperatively) only 13% of the animals were cured. In another study, adriamycin on day 12 and operation on day 15 yielded 65% cures, but with the reverse sequence, i.e., surgery on day 12 and adriamycin on day 15, the cure rate was 47%.

Similar experiments in a different model yielded the same results in BDF1 mice that received implants of Lewis lung tumor. Methyl-CCNU (MeCCNU) given IP on day 7 and surgery on day 8 resulted in 90% cures; the reverse sequence of surgery on day 7 and MeCCNU on day 8 yielded 50% cures (Schabel et al. 1979b). Thus, experimentally, the importance of preoperative chemotherapy in a variety of tumor models and its superiority over postoperative chemotherapy appear to have been well established.

Clinical Studies

Miscellaneous Tumors

In a number of studies chemotherapy alone or as part of multimodality treatment has been used *before* operation with considerable success in a variety of common solid tumors for which surgery was impossible or impractical. In a good many instances surgery has subsequently been feasible and/or more effective. It has been used, for example, in many sarcomas of children and adults (Rivard et al. 1975; Jaffe et al. 1977; Rosen et al. 1976, 1979; Lokich 1979, in nonseminomatous carcinoma of the testes (Merrin et al. 1976; Richie 1978; Vugrin et al. 1981), Wilm's tumor (Sullivan et al. 1967; Wagget and Koop 1970), tumors of the head and neck (Desprez et al. 1970; Tarpley et al. 1975; Elias et al. 1975; Arlen 1976; Frei 1982) lung (Poulsen 1961), and stomach (Rockstroh et al. 1959), adenocarcinoma of the rectum (Wuzoker et al. 1976), squamous cell carcinoma of the anus

(Quan et al. 1978), miscellaneous other solid neoplasms (Avanberg 1964; Kumar et al. 1975; Spanos et al. 1982), and metastatic adenocarcinoma of the liver (Tilchen et al. 1981). Although these studies were not prospective, and usually involved patients with advanced tumors and a dismal prognosis, they nevertheless suggest that this sequence is more effective than the reverse. In none of these studies were any serious problems with wound healing reported.

Breast Cancer

Very few studies of preoperative chemotherapy have been reported to our knowledge, and most have been performed in locally advanced or inflammatory carcinoma. Morris et al. (1978) used combination chemotherapy to treat three patients with metastatic BC who also had locally advanced primary lesions, one with inflammatory BC. Marked regression of the primary sites allowed mastectomies without skin grafts and with no serious postoperative complications. Systemic chemotherapy was continued postoperatively, inducing complete disappearance of distant metastases, and at the time of the report the patients had been clinically free of disease for 21, 10, and 7 months. In nine patients with inflammatory carcinoma (one bilateral) confirmed by thermography but without demonstrable metastases, 9 day polychemotherapy cycles were given monthly until thermographic cooling. Mastectomy followed in six patients, tumorectomies in two, and bilateral tumorectomy in one. Maintenance chemotherapy was given for 1 year and BCG for 3 years. Two patients had local recurrences at 18 and 31 months and were treated by radiotherapy. At the time of this report all patients were in complete remission with survival ranging from 36 to 49 months (Zubberberg et al. 1979).

Preoperative polychemotherapy was also given to 83 patients with locally advanced BC (stages III and IIIc). Shrinkage of the tumor by 50% was observed in 64% of the patients. This effect was less pronounced in 23 patients and no response was seen in 4 patients. This regimen enabled the authors to perform mastectomy in 79 of the 83 patients (Sokolova et al. 1980). Serious postoperative sequelae were not mentioned in any of these reports, but further details are unavailable.

Perioperative Chemotherapy

This group of older studies represents important initial experiments with adjuvant chemotherapy in man. Some of them initially failed to prove their point, although later some long-term benefit was demonstrated. It is of interest that some of them even turned out to be detrimental to patients. In the light of our modern knowledge of tumor kinetics and of host immunity it is important to re-evaluate these initial studies to enable us, in retrospect, to understand and learn from the weaknesses of their design.

The first multicenter trial in the United States of America (Fisher et al. 1968) began in 1958. After radical mastectomy, patients were randomized between placebo and 0.4 mg/kg thio-TEPA IV during surgery and 0.2 mg/kg on days 1 and 2 after the operation. The only group of treated patients in which an effect was demonstrated was that of premenopausal patients with four or more positive nodes. The time to recurrence was 13 months for the placebo group and 45 months for the thio-TEPA group. At 5 years survival in this same subgroup was more than twice as great for the treated as for the placebo group (57% vs 24%, respectively).

It is also interesting that in the overall study there were fewer systemic complications in the thio-TEPA-treated group than in placebo-treated patients. Two postoperative deaths within 30 days occurred, and both patients belonged to the control series.
Nissen-Meyer and his co-workers (1978) in ten collaborating Scandinavian hospitals gave a 6-day course of cyclophosphamide IV on the same day as mastectomy was performed. Radiotherapy followed for all patients. In only one hospital (a radiotherapy clinic) was chemotherapy delayed by 2–4 weeks, because patients were referred there for radiotherapy after mastectomy. Patients in the group receiving cyclophosphamide had a statistically significant reduction in the recurrence rate and an equally significant increase in survival. These differences were greater in patients with more advanced disease and were sustained for up to 15 years (R. Nissen-Meyer, this volume). There was one notable exception in the case of patients who received radiotherapy prior to chemotherapy; in these no benefit was demonstrated, suggesting that the delay of approximately 3 weeks was a crucial factor in this treatment failure. In a trial in England (Finney 1971) in stage I and II patients, cyclophosphamide 2–3 mg/kg IV daily was used, beginning 4 days before simple mastectomy through to the day of operation and for the 5 subsequent days, giving a total dose of 30 mg/kg. Postoperative radiotherapy was administered to all patients. Three years later 18 of 43 treated patients and 25 of 40 controls were disease free, and there had been 22 deaths from cancer in the treated and 13 in the control group. The deaths were in primary stage II patients. The reasons for this effect are not clear. Since the overall dose was small the daily administration and probably the timing may have been sufficiently immunosuppressive to harm treated patients.
In another study in Germany (Rieche et al. 1972), alternate patients with stage I to III disease after radical mastectomy were given 400 mg cyclophosphamide IV on the day of operation and 200 mg daily to a total dose of 1000 mg/kg. Apparently it took 1–2 months for this treatment to be completed. Locoregional recurrence after 3 years was found in 28.4% of controls and 12.2% of treated patients, but this difference was almost exclusively due to reduction of recurrence rates in the group aged 50 years or over. Patients under 50 showed no differences. Among node-positive patients 45.2% of the controls and only 18.1% of treated patients had recurrences at 3 years ($P < 0.1$). The mortality in node-positive patients was 50% and 34.4%, respectively, during the same time. There were no survival differences in the overall group up to 5 years postoperatively, however.
Finally, two studies have been reported from Japan, and very little information is available on the first (Yoshida et al. 1973). After radical mastectomy some of the patients received mitomycin C up to 1 month after operation. At 5 years, survival was 96% for treated patients and 88% for controls. Among node-positive patients, 5-year survival was 86% and 64%, respectively, in those with fewer than three positive nodes; 54% and 44% with three to seven positive nodes; and 20% and 33%, respectively, in patients with more than eight positive nodes. It is not clear, why the patients most at risk (8+ positive nodes) did not respond to this regimen as well as – if not better than – those with fewer positive nodes. The latest study reported from Japan is that of Koyama et al. (1980). Patients randomized to receive chemotherapy were given 0.6 mg/kg mitomycin C divided in to three doses given on the day of mastectomy and in days 3 and 5 thereafter. Cyclophosphamide was given by mouth in doses of 100 mg daily starting 3–4 weeks after operation. The total dose was 21.4 ± 11.8 g given over 9.3 ± 5.8 months. Chemotherapy-treated patients with one to three involved axillary nodes had a 5-year cancer-free survival rate of 84.8%, compared with 57.3% for patients in the control group ($P < 0.05$), and a 5-year cumulative rate of recurrence at distant sites of 5.1%, compared with 31.1% in controls ($P < 0.05$). The effectiveness of chemotherapy was less marked in patients with negative nodes and in those

with four or more positive nodes. Premenopausal patients benefited from chemotherapy more than postmenopausal patients (Koyama et al. 1980). In contrast to the latter Japanese study and the initial NSABP trial mentioned previously, the Scandinavian trial showed equal improvement in premenopausal and postmenopausal patients, suggesting a true chemotherapeutic impact on the disease with that regimen. Although all studies discussed above are concerned with perioperative and not preoperative administration of chemotherapy, they are presented here because they demonstrate the efficacy of systemic therapy when it is used at earlier stages than are usual today. In particular, Nissen-Meyer's work illustrates the importance of timing in adjuvant chemotherapy. A short chemotherapy course that appears effective if begun on the day of mastectomy is entirely ineffective if delayed even by only 3 weeks (Cooper et al. 1982).

Our Own Pilot Studies

We began testing the principle of systemic therapy before operation in a prospective way in October 1976, after an exploratory period, using various drug combinations and schedules in tumors at different sites (Avgoustis et al. 1979). In colorectal tumors, bleeding and obstructive phenomena invariably abated after one 4-day polychemotherapy course with Oncovin, adriamycin, 5-fluorouracil, methotrexate, and cyclophosphamide (Papaioannou et al. 1979). Shrinkage of these tumors was not impressive, however, though some size reduction could often be appreciated by palpation or by endoscopy. Improvement was not conspicious and indeed it was most difficult to estimate, accurately, in the few carcinomas of the gastroesophageal junction, stomach, and pancreas for which preoperative chemotherapy was given. As a result of the chemotherapy-induced decrease in the vascularity of the tumor, regardless of site, a distinct impression was gained in most instances of decreased blood loss and of improved operability. Adverse postoperative sequelae of the healing of abdominal wounds or the intestinal anastomoses were not observed, and systemic postoperative complications were unimpressive. In all our gastrointestinal cases, we have established safety in the performance of surgical interventions, freedom from problems with the operations, and lack of local or systemic complications attributable to the chemotherapy given before operation. Whereas in our initial analysis no differences could be demonstrated between patients treated with polychemotherapy before or after colectomy (Papaioannou et al. 1979), in a more recent analysis with a minimum follow-up of 3 years (Polychronis et al. 1983) the group receiving preoperative chemotherapy with heparin emerged with statistically significantly better survival. In gastric cancer we give 5-fluorouracil, adriamycin, and mitomycin C, 2 weeks before operation (Papaioannou 1981a). The patients, however, are still too few and the time that has passed since the beginning of treatment too short for the impact of this management policy on recurrences or survival to be assessed.

Our Controlled Study in Locally Advanced (Stage III) BC

Taking into account the considerations discussed in the previous sections, the Hellenic Breast Cooperative Group (HBCG) initiated a study using maximal chemoendocrine systemic therapy for the initial assault on locally advanced (stage III) BC (Papaioannou et al. 1983a). It was felt when the protocol was designed that we were justified in making an *initial* all-out effort to treat the systemic disease, which in this group of patients was almost certainly present, even though latent. Systemic therapy was then followed by locoregional treatment. Patients were randomized to receive or not receive postoperative radiotherapy to determine the value of supplementing the initial systemic therapy with maximum (mastectomy and radiotherapy) versus limited (mastectomy only) locoregional treatment.

Patients and Methods

Included in the study were patients up to 75 years of age with tumors 5 cm or greater in the greatest diameter. Patients with fixation of the tumors to the chest wall and redness, peau d'orange, or ulceration over the breast but not exceeding one-third of its surface were also included. More extensive lesions, skin satellites, arm edema, and inflammatory carcinoma were grounds for exclusion. According to the TNM classification of the American Joint Committee and UICC (1977) these categories include all T3 and T4 tumors and some T4b tumors, all N categories but only M0. All patients were required to be generally fit with a Karnofsky performance status > 90% and to have negative posteroanterior and lateral chest x-rays and bone and liver scans. The leukocyte count had to be over 4,000 mm^3 and platelets over 120,000 m^3. Equivocal bone scans constituted a reason for exclusion only if the suggestive areas were verified by appropriate radiographs. Histological diagnosis was established after open biopsy or needle aspiration. Open biopsy performed at another institution was accepted after review of histological sections, but only if protocol treatment could begin within 2 weeks from biopsy. Informed consent was obtained from all patients.

Following stratification according to menopausal status the patients were randomized to group 1 (controls), who underwent mastectomy only, and group 2, who underwent mastectomy and postoperative radiotherapy (study). The premenopausal group included patients whose last menstruation had been 1 year prior to entering the study. All patients received the same 2 day cycles twice before mastectomy: *Day 1,* Oncovin 1.4 mg/m^2, cyclophosphamide 350 mg/m^2, adriamycin 30 mg/m^2; *Day 2,* methotrexate 20 mg/m^2, 5-fluorouracil (5-FU) 350 mg/m^2; all IV and singly. The second cycle was given 3–4 weeks later with the usual hematological precautions. Approximately 30 minutes before anesthesia for mastectomy was initiated, an IV infusion of 5% dextrose in water containing 1000 mg 5-FU was begun. One half of this solution was given during the operation and the remaining half over the ensuing 3–4 hours, so that the entire amount was absorbed over approximately 6 hours. Chemotherapy was resumed about 2 weeks after mastectomy for a total of 12 cycles. However, treatment was withheld for at least 5 weeks in group 2 patients during radiotherapy.

Postmenopausal patients received antiestrogens (20 mg daily) throughout the chemotherapy. Premenopausal patients had bilateral oophorectomy just before mastectomy. The day after mastectomy in all patients a course of antiestrogens 20 mg daily for the entire duration of chemotherapy was started. This medication was taken during radiotherapy in group 2 patients. The protocol designs for premenopausal and postmenopausal patients are presented in Figs. 2 and 3, respectively.

Total mastectomy was required including the pectoralis fascia but not necessarily the pectoralis muscles, with preservation of major nerves and vessels whenever possible and complete axillary dissection. If part or all of the pectoralis muscles or part of the serratous anterior muscle had to be removed this was not considered a protocol violation.

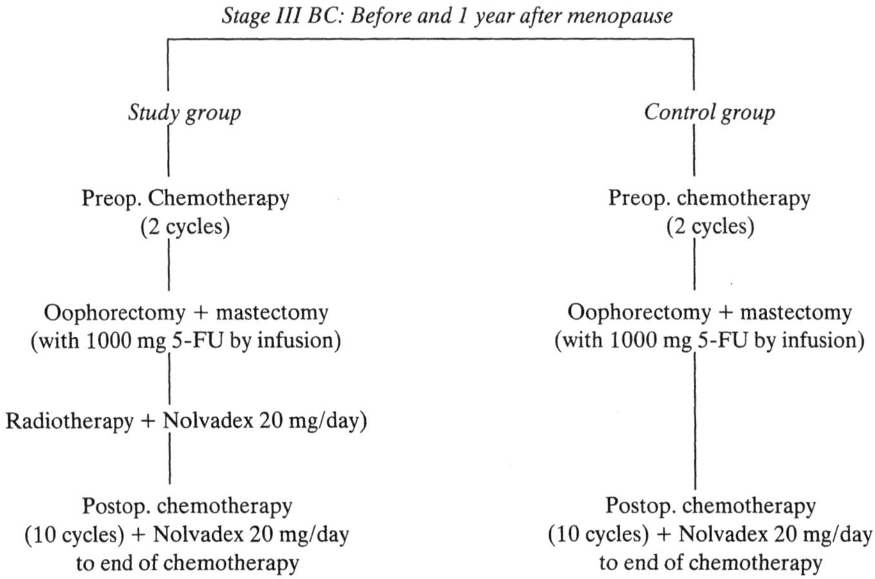

Fig. 2. Protocol design for premenopausal patients

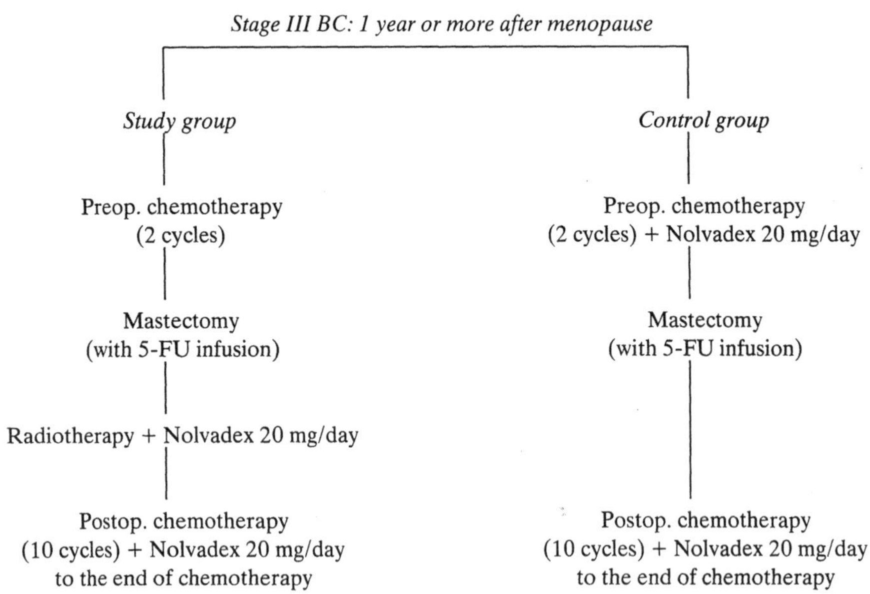

Fig. 3. Protocol design for postmenopausal patients

Patients randomized to radiotherapy received 45–60 Gy to the regional lymph node-bearing areas and chest wall over 5 weeks, beginning 2–3 weeks after operation.

Results

The present analysis refers to 93 patients in group I who had mastectomy only and 92 patients in group 2 who received radiotherapy after mastectomy. These results have been presented elsewhere (Papaioannou et al. 1983b) and are briefly reproduced here. Seventy-eight patients were disqualified. A disproportionately large number of group 2 patients were eliminated because they refused radiotherapy or had other major protocol violations (Table 1). Ultimately 57 patients were evaluable in group 1 and 48 in group 2. Evaluable patients were basically comparable in the two groups in terms of age, mean follow-up, and extent of disease as estimated by the number of positive axillary lymph nodes. Except for the fact that postmenopausal control patients were significantly older than their counterparts receiving radiotherapy, differences were not significant. However,

Table 1. Disqualifications from study by reason in irradiated and nonirradiated groups

Reasons for disqualification	Group	
	1 (No RT)	2 (RT)
Treated elsewhere after 1st or 2nd chemotherapy course	14	15
Had no radiotherapy	–	14
Upstaged (to IV) before or at oophorectomy	5	3
Followed elsewhere after mastectomy	3	–
Did not continue chemotherapy	4	8
Other major protocol violations[a]	6	1
Lost to follow-up	3	2
Died of toxicity after 2nd cycle of chemotherapy	1	–
Total	36	43

[a] The biopsy specimens of two patients were benign. One patient each had oophorectomy prior to entering the study; refused to have chemotherapy for 6 months after mastectomy and later returned; refused to have oophorectomy and had radiation castration in lieu; had previously been treated for carcinoma of the large bowel

Table 2. Comparability of groups

Group	1 (No RT) ($n = 57$)	2 (RT) ($n = 48$)
Mean age	57 years	54.8 years
Mean follow-up	23.6 months	22 months
LN+O	22.3%	18.6%
1–3	25%	30.2%
4+	63.6%	51.1%

group I (controls) was weighted with a greater number of patients with 4+ positive nodes and a smaller percentage of patients with negative nodes than group 2 (Table 2). Crude survival was estimated by the life-table method (Fig. 4) and recurrence-free survival (Fig. 5). Postmenopausal patients fared better in both groups. Those in the control group did better initially but the difference later vanished. The local recurrence rate was higher in premenopausal patients in the control group, whereas systemic recurrences were more frequent in both pre- and postmenopausal patients in the irradiated group, but this difference did not reach statistical significance (Table 3).

Table 4 shows the dissease-free survival of patients who ultimately developed recurrence and Table 5, their length of survival from treatment to death or to the time of the last observation. Control patients (not irradiated) had a longer disease-free survival and a

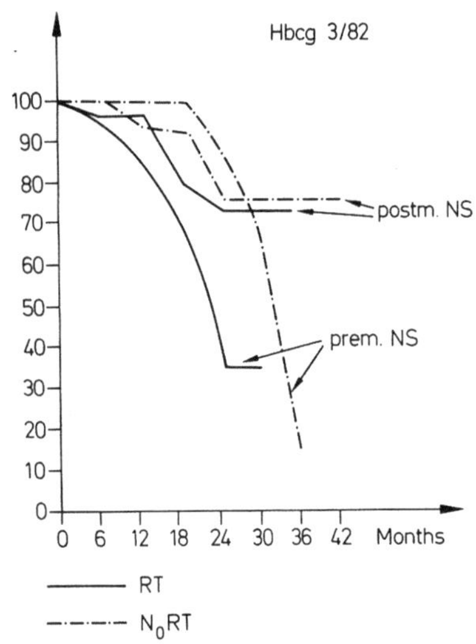

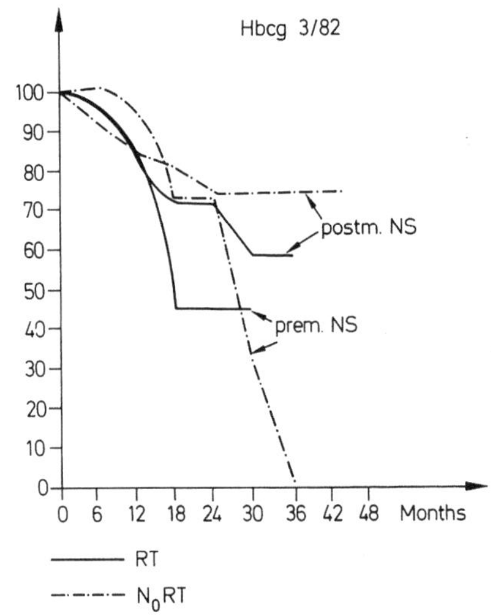

Fig. 4 (*left*). Life-table analysis of crude survival. *NS*, Not significant

Fig. 5 (*right*). Life-table analysis of disease-free survival. *NS*, Not significant

Table 3. Incidence and type of recurrence

Group	1 (No RT) Patients with recurrence (total)	%	2 (RT) Patients with recurrence (total)	%	*P*
Local Premenopausal	2 (19)	10.5	0 (14)	–	NS
Postmenopausal	4 (38)	10.5	4 (34)	11.7	NS
All local	6 (57)	10.5	4 (48)	8.3	NS
Systemic Premenopausal	4 (19)	21	4 (14)	28.5	NS
Postmenopausal	2 (38)	5.3	5 (34)	14.7	NS
All systemic	6 (57)	10.5	9 (48)	18.7	NS
All failures	12 (57)	21	13 (48)	27	NS

NS, Not significant

Table 4. Survival from treatment to recurrence

	1 No RT ($n = 57$)		2 RT ($n = 48$)		P
	Patients	Recurrence (months)	Patients	Recurrence (months)	
Premenopausal	6	26.5	4	14.8	< 0.05
Postmenopausal	6	13.8	9	18.6	> 0.05
Total	12	20.1	13	17.4	> 0.1

Table 5. Total survival from treatment to death (TDD) of patients with recurrence only

Group	1 No RT ($n = 57$)		2 RT ($n = 48$)		P
	Patients	TDD	Patients	TDD	
Premenopausal	6	33.2	4	17.2	< 0.01
Postmenopausal	6	13.8	9	23.7	NS
Total	12	28.7	13	21.7	< 0.05

Table 6. Lymph node involvement in patients with recurrence only

Group	1 No RT ($n = 12$)	2 RT ($n = 13$)
	p : f	p : f
Premenopausal	8.3 : 18	8 : 16
Postmenopausal	10 : 15	7 : 16.6
Total	9.4 : 16.5	7.5 : 16.4

p, positive nodes counted (mean number); f, total number of lymph nodes found (mean)

longer overall survival than their irradiated counterparts. The differences were primarily due to better survival among the premenopausal patients in both instances. Premenopausal patients in the control group who developed recurrences lived approximately 7 months longer free of disease and 16 months longer to death than the corresponding irradiated patients. Both these differences were significant. It seemed possible that the prolonged survival of control patients was not due to the type of therapy used but to differences in the stage of disease prior to radiotherapy. All patients with recurrence were therefore compared for lymph node status (Table 6): Both groups had very advanced disease, but if anything control patients had a higher incidence of positive lymph nodes. The longer survival in patients with recurrent disease must therefore be attributed to the treatment and not to the stage of disease. Postoperative complications were trivial.

Local complications of radiotherapy were also trivial, but moderate myelotoxicity was observed in 15% of these patients, delaying chemotherapy by up to 1 month. On the other hand, nausea, anorexia, and vomiting were invariably observed after each cycle and usually lasted for 2–3 days. Mild myelotoxicity was seen in approximately 80% of patients in both groups. Postponement of the ensuing cycle because of moderate myelotoxicity was necessary more frequently in group 1, particularly in the period of postoperative chemotherapy cycles (Table 7). On the other hand in 80% of patients in group 2 one or more chemotherapy cycles had to be delayed by up to 2 weeks, particularly after radiotherapy.

Discussion

Preoperative systemic therapy is the main treatment modality and the major departure from traditional management in this protocol. However, the study was not designed to evaluate the possible superiority of this over previous treatment methods. The trial design was set up to identify benefits from the addition of aggressive versus limited locoregional treatment to the initial intensive systemic therapy. Hormone receptor analyses were not possible at the initiation of the study and were not therefore taken into consideration in the design of the protocol. It was found that postmenopausal patients generally do better than younger women, particularly if they are not irradiated. Nonirradiated premenopausal patients initially fared better than those who were irradiated, but this effect was later obliterated. With the exception of premenopausal irradiated patients, none of whom has developed recurrence at the time of writing, local disease was equally well controlled in the two groups. Although systemic recurrences in the control group were considerably fewer than in irradiated patients, the inherent aggressiveness of their disease was greater, as evidenced by a smaller percentage of node-negative patients (Table 6) and higher proportion of patients with four or more positive nodes. Also, patients receiving radiotherapy who ultimately relapsed tended to have a shorter disease-free period (Table 4) as well as shorter overall survival (Table 5) than nonirradiated patients. Various reasons can be proposed for the poorer systemic disease control in irradiated patients. The first postoperative chemotherapy cycle began approximately 5–6 weeks later in irradiated patients than in their nonirradiated controls. Further delays of chemotherapy cycles as a result of myelotoxicity were more frequent among irradiated patients (Table 7). Since the dose was held constant in our study, the delays in administering chemotherapy became significant in patients receiving radiotherapy (Table 7). Particularly the initial delay of chemotherapy after mastectomy may be of substantial importance for the systemic component of the disease, which may become enhanced as a result of surgical stress and other tumor-enhancing factors at work in the perioperative period, as discussed in the *Introduction*. An additional factor is that systemic immunity may become depressed after

Table 7. Intervals between chemotherapy cycles

	Group 1 (No RT) $n = 57$	Group 2 (with RT) $n = 48$	Statistical significance
Not completing chemotherapy	7	4	–
Evaluable	50	44	–
Mean interval between postoperative (cycles)	29.14 ± 4.83	34.47 ± 6.55	$P < 0.001$

mediastinal radiotherapy, resulting in decreased survival of the irradiated patients. This has been shown in 8 of 10 controlled trials assessing the value of adjuvant postoperative chemotherapy (Stjernswärd 1977). These detrimental effects of postoperative radiotherapy were recently shown to be more pronounced in patients with regionally advanced but resectable disease, whose need for systemic chemotherapy is obsiously greater (Holland et al. 1980; Cooper et al. 1981; McDonald et al. 1976; Abu-Zahra et al. 1982; Howard et al. 1982).

Detrimental effects of postoperative radiotherapy alone (not combined with chemotherapy) on patients with known or presumed positive nodes were detected (a) in the Cancer Research Campaign trial where radiotherapy, while decreasing local recurrences, in fact increased the mortality rate by 10% in the first year after treatment in documented node-positive patients (Baum and Coyle 1977); (b) in the NSABP protocol No. B-04, in which a wait-and-see policy instead of irradiation appeared to be beneficial in patients with central and inner quadrant lesions, where the incidence of unrecognized internal mammary lymph node chain metastases is highest and theoretically radiotherapy is most needed (Fisher et al. 1981). Furthermore, it has more recently been found that postoperative prophylactic radiotherapy considerably lowers the 5- and 10-year survival of patients with clinical stage II or III BC but negative nodes (Nevin et al. 1982).

The high projected disease-free survival shown in this study (Figs. 4 and 5) is on average threefold higher than that of previously reported series of similar patients treated with preoperative radiotherapy (Whitaker and Battersby 1977; Terz et al. 1978). If this benefit is sustained on longer follow-up, it will corroborate the notion that effective systemic therapy as the initial assault on this disease may be a more appropriate strategy than the reverse therapy sequence (Papaioannou 1980).

As elaborated above, an important conceptual advantage of preoperative chemotherapy is its possible use as a simple, fast, and inexpensive in vivo test of chemosensitivity of the tumor to the drugs used. This hypothesis has now been tested in the same group of stage III BC patients receiving two cycles of preoperative chemotherapy. A detailed analysis of the results of that study has been presented elsewhere (Papaioannou et al. 1983b). Preliminary conclusions from that study are:

1. At 2 weeks after the second chemotherapy course primary tumors had decreased by 25% of their original size in 21% of the patients, by 25%–50% in 34% of the patients, and by more than 50% in 45% of all patients.
2. Tumors of postmenopausal patients responded better than those of younger women. This observation, however, may not be entirely valid, since postmenopausal patients received antiestrogens in addition to preoperative chemotherapy. Clones of hormone-sensitive cells may therefore have responded concomitantly with chemosensitive subpopulations to give a heightened response of primary tumors in older women. This is not unlikely, in view of the usually higher incidence of hormone receptor-positive patients after the menopause (McGuire et al. 1978).
3. Premenopausal patients in whom response was poor had a high probability of recurrence.
4. No relationship could be established between primary tumor shrinkage and subsequent recurrence in postmenopausal patients. The prognostic significance of primary tumor shrinkage following chemotherapy appears therefore to be of clinical value only in poorly responding premenopausal patients.
5. All these conclusions must be considered tentative for the moment, until confirmed by longer follow-up and the study of patients with disease in different stages.

Concluding Comments

Is preoperative chemotherapy going to make a substantial difference to the course of stage III BC? Although our early analysis seems to suggest that this is so, it will take some time before we can be certain of this. As mentioned in the section *Prevention of Development of Drug-Resistant Clones,* the probability of development of chemoresistent cells will change from low to high relatively early in the biological course of the disease (Goldie and Goldman 1979. Taking this into account, if chemotherapy is begun at a late stage, cure of micrometastases may be precluded irrespective of a possible impressive reduction in size of the primary tumor after chemotherapy. Even if this is so, it is not unlikely that preoperative chemotherapy will be considerably more successful in patients in earlier stages of the disease, where both the overall tumor burden and the chances that chemoresistent clones are present are much smaller. Our group is currently studying this point in stage II BC. The evidence reviewed here, however, strongly underscores the importance of early initiation of systemic therapy. Whether or not the ideal time for systemic treatment is before, during, or after surgery remains to be determined. It seems almost certain, however, that systemic treatment begun earlier than is usual today holds considerable promise. In view of our inability to detect and study the behavior of micrometastases in man, the designs of clinical trials testing new hypotheses will necessarily be heavily influenced by the evidence available from animal experimentation. The studies presented in the section on *Experimental Data,* above, are convincing in this regard. To the extent that previous experience in humans is available, it corroborates the impression that the perioperative period is an important phase in the biology of the tumor. If micrometastatic enhancement in fact occurs, as depicted in Fig. 1, therapeutic efforts counteracting this short-lived event may be of greater ultimate value to the patients than much more elaborate systemic therapy beginning 3 weeks later, irrespective of its duration. The Scandinavian success with a 6-day cyclophosphamide course (Nissen-Meyer et al. 1978) can be interpreted on that basis. The same may hold true for the much more limited benefit from the initial NSABP study of thio-TEPA (Fisher et al. 1968) and from the German cyclophosphamide (Rieche et al. 1972) and the Japanese mitomycin C and cyclophosphamide (Koyama et al. 1980) studies discussed above, despite suboptimal drug doses used in all studies.

To our knowledge, in only one instance has concern been expressed about treating micrometastatic disease before the primary tumor is dealt with, by Piro and Hellman (1978). They argue that since some experimental studies suggest that distant metastases may be enhanced by surgery, radiotherapy, or chemotherapy alike, so long as the primary tumor has not been previously treated effectively, viable cell seeding in the immediate posttreatment period may lead to stimulation rather than elimination of metastatic disease. We can perceive little real cause for concern on this point, for the following reasons:

1. In most experimental studies viable cells are infused, usually in large numbers, which does not parallel the human situation.
2. The source of viable cells with the potential to form metastases in man is the primary tumor (Fidler and Kripke 1977). For reasons elaborated above, if the primary tumor is effectively prepared for resection or irradiation by preoperative systemic treatment, intraoperative seeding of cells will be rendered entirely inconsequential.
3. Treatment of primary tumors by chemotherapy before surgery (or radiotherapy) has in fact repeatedly been shown to be of marked benefit in a variety of human tumors (cf. sections: *Miscellaneous Tumors* and *Breast Cancer).*

As previously argued (Papaioannou 1981b) it appears that early systemic treatment is not only appropriate against the systemic component of the disease, but for the initial management of the primary focus as well.

Summary

Many lines of evidence support the view that BC is all too often a systemic disease and that micrometastases become enhanced after resection of the primary. Assuming that these two basic considerations do in fact apply, it can be argued that systemic treatment as the initial attack against operable BC has several advantages over the conventional postoperative adjuvant therapy: (a) Systemic treatment before operation may destroy clonogenic cells in the primary tumor which are responsible for the development of metastases; (b) primary tumor shrinkage following systemic therapy may serve as an early, simple, and inexpensive index of the overall chemosensitivity of the tumor; (c) systemic treatment as soon as the diagnosis is made may prevent the development of drug-resistant mutations, which are likely to form spontaneously early in the natural history of the disease; (d) preoperative chemotherapy may suppress the production of tumor-elaborated substances that protect the tumor from immune destruction by the host; (e) the average delay of about 1 month in the treatment of micrometastases in the postoperative adjuvant setting leads to at least a 30% increase of micrometastatic tumor burden, which can be prevented by preoperative treatment; (f) a number of other considerations suggest that the maximal chemosensitivity of each tumor exists at the earliest possible point in time, i.e., at the time of diagnosis; (g) after the initial postchemotherapy immunosupression immunity recovers, in fact exceeding the pretreatment level, and if surgery is performed during this phase of heightened immunity chemotherapy is utilized as an immunostimulating agent; and finally (h) as more effective systemic agents are discovered, locoregional treatment with surgery and/or radiotherapy may become progressively more limited and it may ultimately be possible to dispense with these modalities.

Experimental evidence scattered in the literature over the past three decades attests to the value of preoperative chemotherapy. Likewise, progressively greater numbers of uncontrolled studies have found preoperative chemotherapy most rewarding in miscellaneous sarcomas and in advanced tumors of the head and neck, kidney, and testes, as well as in a variety of other sites, including the breast. Tests of adjuvant systemic therapy began with a variety of drugs and different perioperative schedules in cooperative multicenter trials as long as 25 years ago. The most successful of these studies is the Scandinavian trial, in which a 6-day cyclophosphamide course beginning on the day of mastectomy conferred significantly better survival in treated premenopausal and postmenopausal patients, which was sustained over 12 years. If the course was delayed by 3 weeks the benefit was no longer evident, suggesting that the timing of chemotherapy, in the immediate postoperative period, was probably the most important component of the study design.

On the basis of the previously mentioned experimental and clinical evidence, we began testing a variety of preoperative chemotherapy schedules for primary operable tumors at miscellaneous sites, including the breast. All regimens given 2–3 weeks before operation were free of operative or postoperative sequelae. When the safety of this policy was established a prospective study was begun by the Hellenic Breast Cooperative Group in July 1978. Patients with clinical stage III BC were given two cycles of 2 day polychemotherapy courses with (per m^2) *Day 1,* Oncovin 1.4 mg, cyclophosphamide 350 mg, and adriamycin 30 mg; *day 2,* methotrexate 20 mg, 5-fluorouracil 350 mg.

Postmenopausal patients received concomitant antiestrogens (20 mg Nolvadex). About 3 weeks after the second cycle mastectomy was performed. The patients were then randomized to receive or not receive radiotherapy (50 Gy) to the chest wall and regional lymphatics over 5 weeks. Premenopausal patients also had oophorectomy on the same day as mastectomy. Postoperative chemotherapy was resumed as soon as possible after mastectomy or radiotherapy. Ten additional cycles were given at intervals of 3–4 weeks. All patients also received Nolvadex 20 mg daily to the end of chemotherapy. Local recurrences were more frequent in premenopausal controls, but systemic dissemination was more frequent in both pre- and postmenopausal irradiated patients. Although this study was not designed to examine the possible superiority of preoperative chemotherapy over conventional policies the projected (actuarial) survival in this series is considerably higher than that achieved in studies with preoperative radiotherapy. Postmenopausal patients fared better in general than younger women. Nonirradiated patients had a longer disease-free survival and a longer overall survival (with disease) than irradiated patients, even though the latter had a slightly lower incidence of positive lymph nodes. The reasons for these detrimental effects of radiotherapy are briefly discussed. Postchemotherapy shrinkage of the primary tumor was more impressive among older than younger women. Correlations with recurrence, however, could be established only in premenopausal women whose tumors responded minimally; this group had the highest probability of recurrence. The development of chemoresistent clones, the probability of which rises from low to high early in the course of the disease, may preclude "cure" if chemotherapy is begun at a late clinical stage. This will be so even in the presence of an impressive shrinkage of the primary tumor in response to chemotherapy. This is why systemic treatment should be progressively more successful, if used in early stages of the evolution of BC. At least in theory, this is exactly the case with preoperative chemotherapy: in each patient treatment begins as soon as possible after the diagnosis is made, thus affording the best chance for cure.

Appendix 1. Participating Services

	Hospital	Responsible surgeon	Responsible chemotherapist	Responsible radiotherapist
Athens	Marika Iliadi	S. Vasilaros	S. Tsiliakos	J. Sakellaris
	IKA	X. Yiotis	S. Tsiliakos	
	Evangelismos Surgical Unit B	A. Papaioannou	K. Alexopoulos	
	Alexandre			K. Papavasiliou
Piraeus	Surgical Unit A DTIP	B. Lissaios	D. Razis	D. Throuvalas
	Surcical Unit B DTIP	V. Georgoulis	D. Razis	D. Throuvalas
	Cynecological DTIP	G. Papadimitriou	D. Razis	D. Throuvalas
	General State Hospital Surgical Unit B	G. Miligos	D. Razis	D. Throuvalas

Statistics: Athens School of Hygiene: G. Papaevangelou, Professor of Hygiene and Biostatistics
Computer Center: Evangelismos Medical Center: Ch. Tsarouhas

References

Abu-Zahra H, McDonald B, Maws J, Mok G, Yoshida S (1982) Effect of adjuvant radiotherapy and chemotherapy in operable cancer of the breast. Presented at the annual meeting of the American Society of Clinical Oncology, April 25, St. Louis

Ader R (1980) Psychosomatic and psychoimmunologic research. Psychosom Med 42: 307–321

Arlen M (1976) Combined radiation methotrexate therapy in preoperative management of carcinoma of the head and neck. Am J Surg 132(4): 536–540

Avanberg S (1974) The effect of preoperative combined bleomycin and radiation therapy in hilar bronchial carcinoma. Scand J Respir Dis [Suppl] 85: 124–133

Avgoustis A, Stathopoulos G, Polychronis A, Papaioannou A (1979) Preoperative chemotherapy of gastrointestinal tumors. A feasibility study. In: Fox IBW (ed) Basis for Cancer therapy. Pergamon, Oxford, pp 263–268

Baum M, Coyle PJ (1977) Simple mastectomy for early breast cancer and the behavior of the untreated axillary nodes. Bull Cancer (Paris) 64: 603–610

Bodgen AE, Esher HJ, Taylor DJ, Gray JH (1974) Comparative study on the effects of surgery chemotherapy and immunotherapy alone and in combination on metastases of the 13762 mammary adenocarcinoma. Cancer Res 34: 1627–1631

Broder S, Waldman TA (1978) The suppressor-cell network in cancer. N Engl J Med 299: 1335–1341

Brock N (1959) Neue experimentelle Ergebnisse mit N-lost-phosphamidestern. Strahlentherapie 41: 347–354

Burchenal JH (1976) Adjuvant therapy theory, practice and potential. The James Ewing Lecture, Cancer 37: 46–57

Cooper MR, Phyne Al, Muss HB and collaborating investigators (1981) A randomized comparative trial of chemotherapy and irradiation therapy for stage II breast cancer. Cancer 47: 2833–2839

Cooper R, Muss H, Feree C, Richards F II, Stuart J, White D, Wells B, Case D, Spurr C (1982) Long-term evaluation of a randomized adjuvant study of chemotherapy (CT) withand without radiation therapy (RT) for stage II breast cancer. Presented at the 5th Annual breast cancer symposium nov. 5–6. Breast Cancer Res Treat 2: 294 (abstr. 72)

Currie GA, Alexander P (1974) Spontaneous shedding of TSTA by viable sarcoma cells. Its possible role in facilitating metastatic spread. Br J Cancer 29: 72–75

Desprez JD, Kiehn CL, Sciotto C, Ramirez-Gonzales M (1970) Response of oral carcinoma to preoperative methotrexate infusion therapy. Am J Surg 120(4): 461–465

DeWys WD (1972) Studies correlating the growth rate of a tumor andits metastases and providing evidence for tumor-related systemic growth retarding factors. Cancer Res 32: 374–379

Elias EG, Shykla SJ, Mink IB (1975) Heparin and chemotherapy in the management of inoperable lung carcinoma. Cancer 36: 129–136

Fidler JJ, Kripke ML (1977) Metastasis results from pre-existing variant cells within a malignant tumor. Science 197: 893–895

Finney R (1971) Adjuvant chemotherapy in the radical treatment of carcinoma of the breast. A clinical trial. AJR 111: 137–141

Fisher B (1977) Biological and clinical considerations regarding the use of surgery and chemotherapy in the treatment of primary breast cancer. Cancer 40: 574–587

Fisher B, Ravdin RG, Ausman RK, Slack NH, Moore GE, Noer RJ and cooperating investigators (1968). Surgical adjuvant chemotherapy in cancer of the breast: results of a decade of cooperative investigations. Ann Surg 168: 337–356

Fisher B, Gebhardt M, Saffer E (1979) Further observations on the inhibition of tumor growth by C Parvum with cyclophosphamide: VII effect of treatment prior to primary tumor removal on the growth of distant tumor. Cancer 43: 451–458

Fisher B, Wollmack N, Redmond C, Deutsch M, Fisher E and participating NSABP investigators (1981) Findings from NSABP protocol no. B-04. Comparison of radical mastectomy with

alternative treatments II. The clinical and biologic significance of medial-central breast cancer. Cancer 48: 1863–1872
Folkman J, Cotran R (1976) Relation of vascular proliferation to tumor growth. Int Rev Exp Pathol 16: 207–248
Frei E III (1977) Rationale for combined therapy. Cancer 40: 569–573
Frei E III (1982) Clinical cancer research. An embattled species. Cancer 50: 1979–1992
Goldie JH, Coldman AJ (1979) A mathematical model for relating the drug sensitivity of tumors to their spontaneous mutation rate. Cancer Treat Rep 63: 1727–1733
Gorelik E, Segal S, Feldman M (1978) Growth of a local tumor exerts a specific inhibitory effect on progression of lung metastases. Int J Cancer 21: 617–625
Gunduz N, Fisher B, Saffer E (1979) Effect of surgical removal on the growth and kinetics of residual tumor. Cancer Res 39: 3861–3865
Harris J, Senger D, Stewart T, Hyslop D (1976) The effects of immunosuppressive chemotherapy on immune function in patients with malignant disease. Cancer 37: 1058–1069
Henderson IC, Canellos GP (1980) Cancer of the breast. The past decade. N Engl J Med 302: 17–27
Heuser L, Spratt JS Jr, Polk HC Jr (1979) Growth rates of primary breast cancer. Cancer 43: 1888–1894
Holland JF, Glidewell O, Cooper RG (1980) Adverse effects of radiotherapy on adjuvant chemotherapy for carcinoma of the breast. Surg Gynecol Obstet 150: 817–821
Howard O, Margolski I, Strauss MJ, Ambinder JM, Alvarez E, Diamond R, Madden RE (1982) Adverse effects of RT on chemotherapy dosage in breast cancer adjuvant therapy. Presented at the annual meeting of the American Society of Clinical Oncology, April 25–27, St. Louis
Jaffe N, Frei E III, Traggis D, Watts H (1977) Weekly high-dose methotrexate citrovorum factor in osteogenic sarcoma. Pre-surgical treatment of primary tumor and of overt pulmonary metastases. Cancer 39: 45–50
Kaplan HS, Murphy ED (1948) The effect of local roentgen irradiation on thebiological behavior of a transplantable mouse carcinoma I. Increased frequency of pulmonary metastasis. JNCI 407–413
Karrer K, Humphreys SR, Goldin A (1967) An experimental model for studying factors which influence metastases of malignant tumors. Int J Cancer 2: 213–223
Ketcham AS, Wexler H, Mantel N (1959) The effect of removal of a Primary tumor on the development of spontaneous metastases. I. Development of a standardized experimental technic. Cancer Res 19: 940–944
Ketcham AS, Kinsey DL, Wexler H, Mantel N (1961) The development of spontaneous metastases after removal of a "primary tumor". II: Standardization protocol of five animal tumors. Cancer 14: 875–882
Koyama H, Wada T, Takahashi Y, Nishizawa Y, Iwanaga T, Aoki I, Torarawa T, Kosaki G, Kajita A, Wada A (1980) Surgical adjuvant chemotherapy with Mitomycin C and cyclophosphamide in Japanese patients with breast cancer. Cancer 46: 2373–2379
Kumar APM, Wrenn EL Jr, Felming ID, Hustu HO, Pratt CB, Pinkel DJ (1975) Preoperative therapy for unresectable malignant tumors in children. J Pediatr Surg 10: 567–670
Langlands AO, Pocock SJ, Kerr GR, Gore SM (1979) Long-term survival of patients with breast cancer. A study of the curability of the disease. Br Med J II: 1247–1251
Lokich JJ (1979) Preoperative chemotherapy in soft tissue sarcoma. Surg Gynecol Obstet 148: 512–516
McDonald AM, Simpson JS, McIntyre J (1976) Treatment of early cancer of the breast. Histological staging and role of radiotherapy. Lancet I: 1098–1100
McGuire WL, Horwitz KB, Zava DT, Garola RE (1978) Interpreting data from steroid receptor assays in human breast tissue. Reviews on Endocrine Related Cancer 1: 5–12
McLoughlin GA, Wu AV, Saporoschetz I, Nimberg R, Mannick J (1979) Correlation between anergy and a circulating immunosuppressive factor following major surgical trauma. Ann Surg 190: 297–304

Merrin C, Takita H, Weber R, Wajsman Z, Baumgarden G, Murphy G (1976) Combination radical surgery and multiple sequential chemotherapy for the treatment of advanced carcinoma of the testis (stage III). Cancer 37: 20–29

Miller BE, Miller FR, Leith J, Heppner GM (1980) Growth interaction in vivo between tumor subpopulations derived from a single mouse mammary tumor. Cancer Res 40: 3977–3981

Morris D, Aisner J, Elion EG, Wiernik PH (1978) Mastectomy as an adjuvant to combination chemotherapy. Arch Surg 113: 282–284

Morton DL, Eilber FR, Townsend CM Jr, Grant TT, Mirra J, Weissenburger TH (1976) Limb salvage from a multidisciplinary treatment approach for skeletal and soft tissue sarcomas of the extremity. Ann Surg 184: 268–278

Mueller CB, Ames F, Anderson GB (1978) Breast cancer in 3558 women. Age as a significant determinant in the rate of dying and causes of death. Surgery 83: 123–132

Nealon TF Jr, Nkougho A, Grossi C, Gilloley J (1979) Pathologic identification of poor prognosis stage 1 (T1NoMo) cancer of the breast. Ann Surg 190: 129–132

Nevin JE, Baggerly JT, Kerr Laird D (1982) Radiotherapy as an adjuvant in the treatment of carcinoma of the breast. Cancer 49: 1194–1200

Newberry BH (1981) Effects of presumafly stressful stimulation (PSS) on the development of animal tumors. Some issues. In: Weiss SM, Herd JA, Fox BH (eds) Perspectives on behavioral medicine. Academic, New York, pp 329–349

Nissen-Meyer R, Kjellgren K, Malmiok K, Mansson B, Norin T (1978) Surgical adjuvant chemotherapy. Results with one short course with cyclophosphamide after mastectomy for breast cancer. Cancer 41: 2088–2098

North RJ, Kirstein DP, Tuttle RL (1976) Subversion of host defense mechanisms by murine tumors I. A circulating factor that surpresses macrophage-mediated resistence to infection. J Exp Med 143: 559–573

Norton L, Simon R (1977) Tumor size, sensitivity to therapy and design of treatment schedules. Cancer Treat. Rep 61: 1307–1317

Osteen RT, Chaffey JT, Moore FD, Wilson RE (1978) An agressive multi modality approach to locally advanced carcinoma of the breast. Surg Gynecol Obstet 147: 75–79

Papaioannou AN (1980) Chemotherapy before mastectomy may be a more effective therapeutic sequence than its reverse in primary operable breast cancer. In: Mouridsen HT, Palshof T (eds) Breast cancer-experimental and clinical aspects. Pergamon, Oxford, pp 255–258

Papaloannou AN (1981a) Why do fall in gastric cancer. What can we do about it? In: Mainz M, Friedman M, Ogawa M, Kisner D (eds) Proceedings of the international congress of diagnosis and treatment of upper-gastrointestinal tumors, Sept. 9–11 1980. Excerpta Medica, Amsterdam, pp 237–252

Papaioannou AN (1981b) Preoperative chemotherapy for operable solid tumors. Eur J Cancer 17: 263–269

Papaioannou AN (1981c) Enhancement by local treatment. In: Stoll B (ed) New aspects in breast cancer, vol 4. Heineman Medical, London, pp 167–187

Papaioannou AN (1982) Informed consent after randomization. (Letter) Lancet II: 828

Papaioannou AN, Urban J (1964) Scalene node biopsy in locally advanced primary cancer of the breast of questionable operability. Cancer 17: 1006–1011

Papaioannou AN, Nomikos J, Stathopoulos G, Avgoustis A, Olympitis J (1979) Pre and postoperative chemotherapy with or without anticoagulation for colorectal cancer. Clin Oncol 5: 189–190

Papaioannou AN, Lissaios B, Vassilaros St, Miligos S, Papadimitriou G, Kondilis D, Polychronis A, Kozonis J, Papageorgiou G, Plataniotis G, Razis D, Stathopoulos G, Tsiliakos St, Papavasiliou K, Throuvalas N, Tsarouhas Ch, Papaevangelou G (1983a) Pre and postoperative chemoendocrine treatment with or without postoperative radiotherapy for locally advanced breast cancer. Cancer 51: 1284–1290

Papaioannou AN, Kozonis J, Polychronis A, Papageorgiou G, Lissaios B, Kondylis D, Vasilaros St, Papadiamantis J, Tsiliakos St, Razis D, Throuvalas N, Papavasiliou K, Sakelaris J, Tsarouhas Ch and collaborating investigators of the Hellenic Breast Cooperative Group (HBCG) (1983b)

Shrinkage of stage III primary breast cancer BC to preoperative (Preop) systemic therapy (RX). Presented to the 3rd EORTC breast cancer working conference, April 28, Amsterdam.
Pearlman NW, Guerra O, Fracchia AA (1976) Primary inoperable cancer of the breast. Surg Gynecol Obstet 143: 909–913
Pendergrast WJ Jr, Drake WP, Mardiney MR Jr (1976) A proper sequence for the treatment of B16 melanoma. Chemotherapy, surgery and immunotherapy. JNCI 57: 539–544
Pike MC, Snyderman R (1976) Depression of macrophage function by a factor produced by neoplasms. A mechanism for abrogation in immune surveillance. J Immunol 117: 1243–1249
Piro AJ, Hellman S (1978) Effect of primary treatment modality on the metastatic pattern of mammary carcinoma. Cancer Treat Rep 62: 1275–1280
Polychronis A, Plataniotis G, Papaioannou A, Coca H, Tsamouri M, Kalapothaki V, Trichopoulos D (1983) Pre-intra and postoperative chemotherapy (CH) with or without anticoagulation in colorectal cancer. ASCO annual meeting, San Diego (abstr. no. C-512)
Poulsen O (1961) Prae- und postoperative cytostatische Behandlung von Lungencarcinomen mit Cyclophosphamid. Arzneimittelforsch 11: 238–242
Quan SHQ, Magill GB, Leaming RH, Hadjo SI (1978) Multidisciplinary preoperative approach to the management of epidermoid carcinoma of the anus and anorectum. Dis Colon Rectum 21: 89–91
Richie JP (1978) Combination chemotherapy and surgery: an aggressive approach to stage III testis tumors. Presented at the 31st annual meeting of the Society of Surgery and Oncology, April 3, San Diego
Rieche K, Berndt H, Prahl B (1972) Continuous postoperative treatment with cyclophosphamide in breast carcinoma. A randomized clinical study. Arch Geschwulstforsch 40: 349–354
Riley V (1981) Psychoneuroendocrine influences on immunocompetence and neoplasia. Science 212: 1100–1109
Rivard G, Ortega J, Hittle R, Nitschke R, Karon M (1975) Intensive chemotherapy as primary treatment for rhabdomyosarcoma of the pelvis. Cancer 36: 1593–1597
Rockstroh H, Hasselbacher K, Barth F (1959) Die Kombinationsbehandlung Krebskranker in der Chirurgie. Pruns Beitr Klin Chir 199: 355–364
Rollinghoff M, Starzinski-Powitz A, Pfizenmaierk (1977) Cyclophosphamide sensitive T lymphocyte suppress the in vivo generation of antigen-specific cytotoxic T lymphocytes. J Exp Med 145: 455–459
Rosen G, Murphy ML, Huvos AG (1976) Chemotherapy, en bloc resection and prosthetic bone replacement in the treatment of osteogenic sarcoma. Cancer 37: 1–11
Rosen G, Marcove RC, Caparros B, Cahill L, Hyvos AG (1978) Primary osteogenic sarcoma. The rationale for treatment with preoperative chemotherapy and delayed surgery. Cancer 41: 841–849
Rosen G, Marcove RC, Caparros B, Nirenberg A, Kosloff C, Huvos AG (1979) Primary osteogenic sarcoma. The rationale for preoperative chemotherapy and delayed surgery. Cancer 43: 2163–2177
Rutqvist LE, Wallgren A (1982) Long-term follow up of 458 young breast cancer patients. Aspects on the curability of the disease. Presented in fundamental problems in breast cancer, Sept. 17–18, Jasper Alberta
Saba TM (1978) Prevention of liver endothelial systemic host defense failure after surgery by intravenous opsonic glycoprotein therapy. Ann Surg 188: 142–152
Schabel FM Jr (1977) Rationale for adjuvant chemotherapy. Cancer 39: 2875–2882
Schabel FM Jr, Griswold DP Jr, Corbett TH, Laster WR Jr, Dykes DJ, Rose WC (1979a) Recent studies with adjuvant chemotherapy or immunotherapy of metastatic solid tumors of mice. In: Jones II SE, Salmon SE (eds) Adjuvant therapy of cancer. Proceedings of the 2nd international conference. Grune and Stratton, New York, pp 476–483
Schabel FM Jr, Corbett TH, Griswold DP Jr, Laster WR Jr, Dykes DJ, Rose WC (1979b) Recent studies with surgical adjuvant chemotherapy or immunotherapy of metastatic solid tumors of mice. In: Jones SE II, Salmon SE (eds) Adjuvant therapy of cancer, vol 2. Grune and Stratton, New York, pp 3–14

Schatton WE (1958) An experimental study of postoperative tumor metastases. I. Growth of pulmonary metastases following total removal of primary leg tumor. Cancer 11: 455–459

Selby P, Buick RN, Tannock I (1983) A critical appraisal of the "human tumor stem-cell assay". N Engl J Med 308: 129–134

Sheldon PW, Fowler JF (1973) The effect of irradiating a transplanted murine lymphosarcoma on the subsequent development of metastases. Br J Cancer 28: 508–514

Sherwin SA, Minna JD, Gazder AF, Todaro GJ (1981) Expression of epidermal and nerve growth factor receptors and soft agar growth factor production by human lung cancer cells. Cancer Res 41: 3538–3542

Simpson-Herren L, Sanford AH, Holmquist JP (1976) Effects of surgery on the cell kinetics of residual tumor. Cancer Treat Rep 60: 1749–1760

Skipper HE, Schabel FM Jr, Wilcox WS (1964) Experimental evaluation of potential anticancer agents. XIII: On the criteria and kinetics associated with "curability" of experimental leukemia. Cancer Chemother Rep 35: 1–111

Sokolova IG, Vishnykova, Soyatukhina OV (1980) Preoperative polychemotherapy in the complex treatment of locally spread cancer of the mammary gland. Vopr Onkol 26: 9–13

Spanos GA, Wolk D, Desner MR, Khan A, Platt N, Khafif RA, Corten EP (1982) Preoperative chemotherapy for giant cell carcinoma of the thyroid. Cancer 50: 2252–2256

Sporn MB, Todaro GJ (1980) Autocrine secretion and malignant transformation of cells. N Engl J Med 303: 878–880

Steel GG (1977) Growth kinetics of tumors. Glarendon, Oxford

Stjernswärd J (1977) Adjuvant radiotherapy trials in breast cancer. Cancer 39: 2846–2851

Sullivan MP, Sutow WW, Cangir A, Taylor G (1967) Vincristine sulfate in management of Wilm's tumor. JAMA 202: 381–384

Tarpley JL, Chretien PB, Alexander JC Jr, Hoye RC, Block JB, Ketcham AS (1975) High dose methotrexate as a preoperative adjuvant in the treatment of epidermoid carcinoma of the head and neck. A feasibility study and clinical trial. Am J Surg 130(4): 481–486

Terz JJ, Romero CA, Kay S, Brown PW, Wassum J, King ER, Lawrence W Jr (1978) Preoperative radiotherapy for stage III carcinoma of the breast. Surg Gynecol Obstet 147: 497–502

Tilchen E, Patt VZ, McBride CM, Wallace S, Chuang V, Mavligit CM (1981) Sequence of regional chemotherapy and surgery. Management of colorectal adenocarcinoma confined to the liver. Ann Surg 116: 959–960

Tyzzer EE (1913) Factors in the production and growth of tumor metastases J Med Res 28: 309–332

Van den Brenk HAS, Sharpington C (1971) Effect of local x-irradiation of a primary sarcoma in the rat on dissemination and growth of metastases. Dose-response characteristics. Br J Cancer 25: 812–830

Von Hoff DD (1983) Send this patient's tumor for culture and sensitivity. N Engl J Med 308: 154–155

Vugrin D, Whitmore WF Jr, Sogani PC, Bains M, Hew HW, Golbey RB (1981) Combined chemotherapy and surgery in treatment of advanced germ-cell tumors. Cancer 47: 2228–2231

Wagget J, Koop CE (1970) Wilms' tumor. Preoperative radiotherapy and chemotherapy in the management of massive tumors. Cancer 26: 338–340

Whitaker SV, Battersby C (1977) The dilema of stage III breast cancer. A study of preoperative radiotherapy. Aust NZ J Surg 47: 684–687

Wuzoker J, Nigro N, Correa J, Vaitkevicius VK, Samson M, Considine B (1976) Combination preoperative radiation and chemotherapy in adenocarcinoma of the rectum. Preliminary report. Dis Colon Rectum 19: 660–663

Yoshida Y, Miura S, Murou H, Takenchi S (1973) Late results of combined chemotherapy for cure of breast cancer (axillary lymph node metastasis and therapeutic effect). In 10th annual meeting of the Japanese Society for Cancer Therapy (abstr. no. 177)

Zacharski LR, Henderson WG, Pickles FR, Forman WB, Cornell CJ Jr, Forcier RJ, Horrower HW, Johnson RO (1979) Rationale and experimental design for the VA cooperative study of anticoagulation in the treatment of cancer. Cancer 44: 732–741

Zubberberg B, Amiel JP, Jamain B, Ponillart P, Ravina JH, Salat-Baront J (1979) Preoperative immunochemotherapy in the treatment of inflammatory breast cancer. Preliminary results of a trial in nine patients. Nouv Presse Med 8: 755–758

Short Perioperative Versus Long-Term Adjuvant Chemotherapy

R. Nissen-Meyer, H. Host, K. Kjellgren, B. Mansson, and T. Norin*

Tyribakken 10, Oslo 2, Norway

Introduction

The Scandinavian Adjuvant Chemotherapy Study Group (Appendix 1) has conducted trials of Chemotherapy in breast cancer, two of which are reported below

First Scandinavian Study

The questions we asked were these:

1. Can one single, short perioperative chemotherapy course increase the ultimate cure rate?
2. Can a delay of a few weeks between mastectomy and the start of chemotherapy reduce the effect?

Some experimental animal studies had indicated these two possibilities, but they had not been demonstrated clearly in clinical studies (Schabel 1977).

Methods

We started our first study in January 1965. In ten surgical clinics operable routine cases were randomized by telephone from the operating theater. The experimental group received cyclophosphamide IV 5 mg/kg daily for 6 days, the first injection being given immediately after mastectomy.

The eleventh hospital participating in the first study was a Radiotherapy Clinic. The patients went to this clinic between 2 and 4 weeks after mastectomy and were randomized after arrival. For experimental group at this hospital there was therefore an interval of about 3 weeks between mastectomy and the start of adjuvant chemotherapy. However, the chemotherapy course was the same in all hospitals, and the patients in all hospitals underwent both mastectomy and postoperative radiotherapy.

---

* For the Scandinavian Adjuvant Chemotherapy Study Group; the members of the Group are listed in Appendix 1

Recent Results in Cancer Research. Vol. 98

Further details of the case material, treatment methods, statistical methods, and immediate side-effects can be found in a previous paper (Nissen-Meyer et al. 1978).

Side-Effects

The immediate side-effects of the short cyclophosphamide course were very moderate, of short duration, and easy to relieve with antiemetic drugs, etc., since during the treatment period the patients were still in hospital after the mastectomy.

There have been some reports in the literature that long-term chemotherapy may induce other malignant diseases after a delay of some 5–10 years (Chabner 1977). We have looked for this possibility in our material, and found 37 cases of secondary leukemia, lymphomas, and carcinomas (Table 1). However, 21 were in the control group, and only 16 in the group with chemotherapy. Accordingly, there is no reason to blame the short cyclophosphamide course. We only observed a general tendency for patients cured from one cancer to develop new malignant diseases.

Results

Figure 1 demonstrates the relapse-free percentages from the ten hospitals where adjuvant chemotherapy was instituted immediately after mastectomy. The difference in favor of the 507 cyclophosphamide cases was small at the beginning, was highly significant by 4 years after mastectomy, and was thereafter maintained at a level of about 12% up to at least 16 years after mastectomy.

This shape of the curves gives no indication that the effect of the short perioperative course might be merely to delay the clinical appearance of metastases. The effect observed is in harmony with a hypothesis of a true increase in ultimate cure rate (Nissen-Meyer 1979).

Subgroup analyses by axillary lymph node status and menopausal status did not reveal a different treatment effect in any of these subgroups.

In Fig. 2 the same two curves are compared with the corresponding curves from the one hospital where the same short cyclophosphamide course was given 2–4 weeks after mastectomy. In this hospital the chemotherapy course apparently had no effect – the curve in both groups is very similar to that in the control group from the ten hospitals with the perioperative course. The chance fluctuations are of course more pronounced in the curves from the smaller groups.

Table 1. Secondary malignant disease observed (excluding mammary and basocellular carcinoma)

	Cyclophosphamide group	Control group
Leukemia	0	1
Lymphomas	2	2
Gynecological cancer	3	6
Gastrointestinal cancer	8	6
Other carcinomas	3	6
Total	16	21

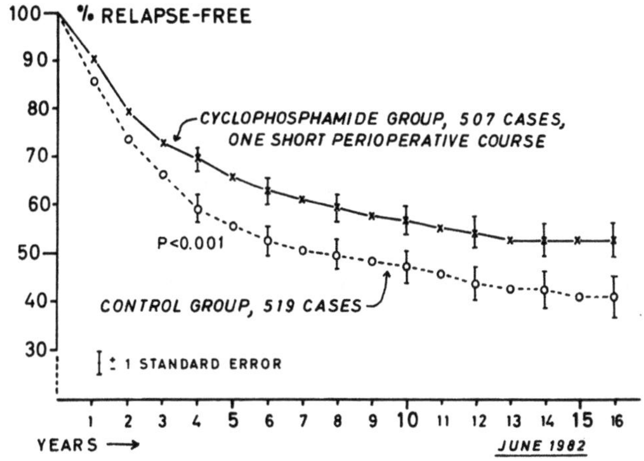

Fig. 1. Results in study 1. The main series with one short perioperative course

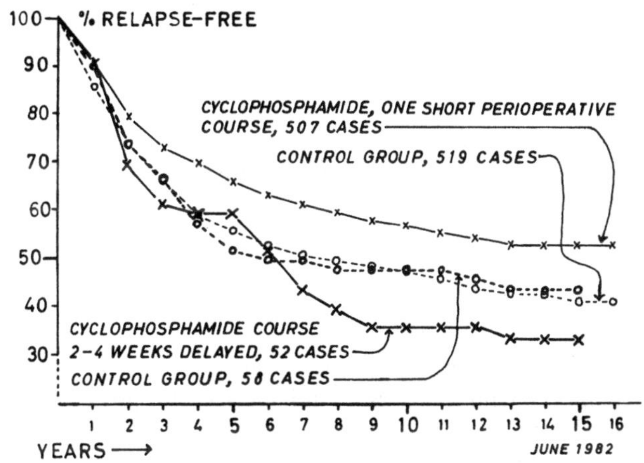

Fig. 2. Results in study 1. A comparison of the delayed course with the perioperative course

Our first study allows the following conclusions:

1. One short chemotherapy course immediately after mastectomy can increase the ultimate cure rate about 12%, with virtually negligible side-effects and with no risk.
2. This treatment schedule seems now indicated in stage I and stage II, in both postmenopausal and premenopausal patients.
3. By 2–4 weeks after mastectomy the optimum time for start of adjuvant chemotherapy may be over.

Second Scandinavian Study

The next question we asked was: Does the benefit accruing from continuing the adjuvant treatment for 1 year justify the increased side-effects and possible risks of long-term chemotherapy?

Methods

In March 1977 we started our second study, in an attempt to answer this question. All our patients now receive one short chemotherapy course immediately after mastectomy.

When the pathologist has finished evaluation of the specimens, the node-positive cases are randomized between an experimental group, in which the patients are to continue with chemotherapy for 1 year, and a control group with no more adjuvant chemotherapy. Node-negative cases receive no further adjuvant chemotherapy.

To date we have 317 node-positive cases and 637 node negative cases. The study is still open.

(One half of all these patients are also randomized to receive immunotherapy with *Corynebacterium parvum* SC around the mastectomy scar. This treatment has had no effect on the overall results so far, and no results will be published before we have collected a reasonable number followed up for 5 years in the various subgroups.)

We modernized the short perioperative course from the single-drug therapy in our first study to a multidrug course; a slight modification of a schedule found in advanced breast cancer to strike a favorable balance between effectiveness and side-effects (Edelstyn et al. 1975).

For long-term chemotherapy we have used CMF given IV on days 1 and 8 of each 4-week cycle for 12 cycles.

The doses for the short perioperative course and the longterm treatment are shown in Table 2.

Side-Effects

The short perioperative multidrug course has been as well tolerated as the short cyclophosphamide course, and caused no problems. We have now used it in 954 cases.

The side-effects of the long-term CMF treatment have been a major problem, both for the patients and for ourselves.

Only 37% of the patients managed to complete this treatment with at least 90% of the scheduled dose. In one-half of these cases the treatment was considered fairly well

Table 2. Chemotherapy schedules in study 2

	Short perioperative course		CMF for 1 year	
	Day 0	Day 7	Day 1	Day 8
Cyclophosphamide IV	500 mg	500 mg	500 mg	500 mg
Vincristine IV	1 mg	1 mg	–	–
5-FU IV	750 mg	–	750 mg	750 mg
Methotrexate IV	–	50 mg	50 mg	50 mg
	Only one course		Repeated every 4 weeks	

The doses above are referred to 70 kg; doses are adjusted according to body weight

tolerated. The other half suffered considerably from the side-effects, mainly nausea and vomiting, which could continue for a whole week after each injection. A reduction of the doses had little effect on these side-effects.
The first few courses were usually not so bad, but nausea and vomiting subsequently tended to increase in severity from course to course, and 38% of the patients eventually insisted that the treatment should be terminated, after a median of 14 injections.
This must necessarily reduce the chances of an effective secondary treatment of recurrent disease. The patients who have once learned to hate cytotoxic drugs hardly ever forget it!
The possible late complications of long-term chemotherapy in this study are still unknown, but secondary malignancies can be expected to occur.

Results

Figure 3 shows the percentages of node-negative cases that were relapse-free in both studies. The results in study 2 are only slightly better than those obtained in the experimental group of study 1, suggesting that the new multidrug perioperative course is about as effective as the earlier cyclophosphamide course was.
Figure 4 shows the percentages of node-positive cases that were relapse-free in both studies. The results in the control group of study 2 are slightly better than those in the experimental group of study 1, suggesting again that the new multidrug perioperative course is at least as effective as the earlier single-drug therapy.
The effect of prolonging adjuvant treatment with chemotherapy for 1 year is reflected in the difference between the two curves recorded in study 2. Or rather, this is the effect of our intention to continue adjuvant chemotherapy for 1 year. A clear decision on the part of the patient to terminate the treatment must be respected.
After 1 year there is a difference of 10.1% ($P < 0.05$). Beyond this point, so far we have followed up too few cases for a reliable assessment of the results. The continued follow-up, however, may give us a better indication as to whether the additional effect of the prolonged chemotherapy is really an additionally increased cure rate, or merely a delay in clinical appearance of the recurrent disease.

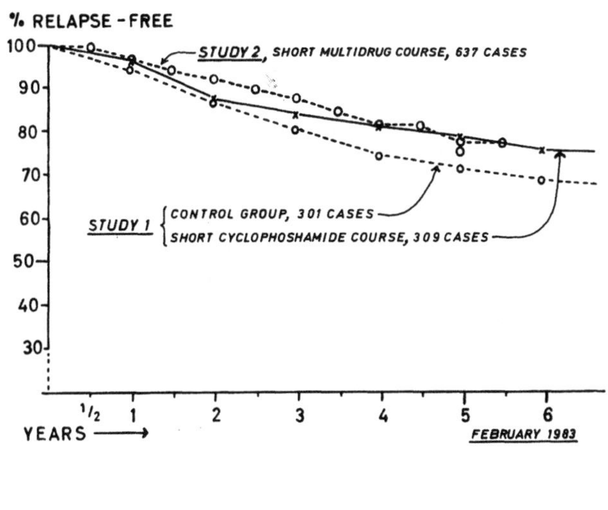

Fig. 3. Results in stage I disease in node-negative cases. A comparison of study 2 with study 1

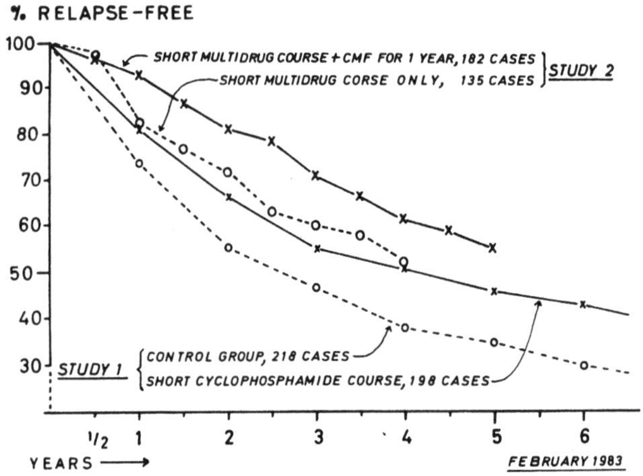

Fig. 4. Results in stage II disease in node-positive cases. A comparison of study 2 with study 1

Discussion

The justification for all types of adjuvant treatment should be assessed after a careful evaluation of the factors shown in Fig. 5.

The value of any particular treatment modality depends on its ability to increase the cure rate and to delay the onset of clinically evident disease. Of these two factors an increased ultimate cure rate should be given a considerably heavier weighting than a simple delay of clinical disease.

Factors that count as negative features of a treatment are the risks it entails and side-effects. We are now paying much more attention to the influence on the quality of life than we did some years ago.

We must also bear in mind that only the patients not cured by the mastectomy alone will benefit from the adjuvant treatment, whereas all patients treated are exposed to the risks and side-effects.

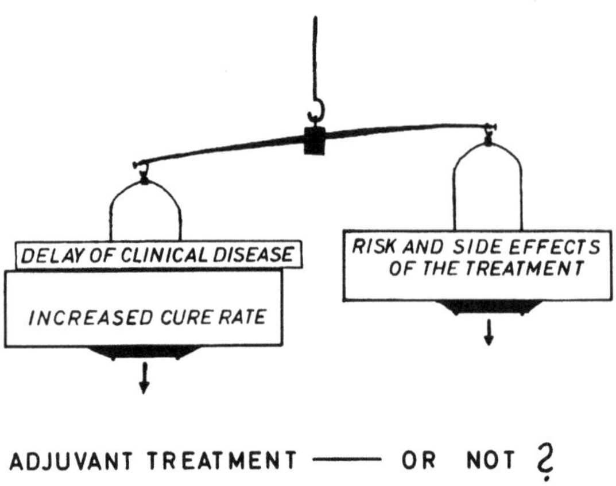

Fig. 5. Essential factors in the decision for or against adjuvant therapy

This means that on the balance the effect of a treatment must be very favorable to justify its use in low-risk cases, whereas it seems more reasonable to accept more severe side-effects in high-risk cases.
The virtually insignificant side-effects and apparent absence of risk in the case of the short perioperative course means that this treatment schedule is justified even in low-risk cases.
Our material does not yet allow us to draw any firm conclusions about the justification of the long-term CMF schedule we are trying, but its unfavorable influence on the quality of life throughout the treatment period makes it obviously unsuitable for use in low-risk cases.
The side-effects increased in severity with increasing duration of the chemotherapy. Many more, and larger, trials are obviously needed to find the optimum duration of adjuvant chemotherapy taking into account of both benefit and side-effects.

Summary

A single course of cyclophosphamide IV 5 mg/kg daily for 6 days was given immediately after mastectomy to 507 patients (519 randomized controls). The relapse-free rates were significantly increased, and after 16 years the difference was 12%.
In a parallel series the same adjuvant course was given 2–4 weeks after mastectomy to 52 patients (58 randomized controls). No effect of this delayed course was found.
In a second study a short multidrug course was given to all patients immediately after mastectomy. One-half of the axillary node-positive cases were randomized to continue with IV CMF for 1 year. The preliminary observations show that the prolonged treatment improved the relapse-free rates significantly during the first few years. One year after mastectomy the difference was 10%; after 2 years, 9%; after 3 years, 11%; and after 4 years, 9%.
The side-effects of the short course were negligible, but the side-effects of prolonged treatment were considerable and increased with increasing treatment duration.
More trials are needed to find the optimum duration of adjuvant chemotherapy.

References

Chabner BA (1977) Second neoplasm – a complication of cancer chemotherapy. N Engl J Med 297: 213–215

Edelstyn GA, Bates TD, Brinkley D, MacRae KD, Spittle MF, Wheeler T (1975) Comparison of 5-day, 1-day, and 2-day cyclical combination chemotherapy in advanced breast cancer. Lancet 2: 209–211

Nissen-Meyer R (1979) Adjuvant cytostatic and endocrine therapy: increased cure rate or delayed manifest disease. In: Bulbrook RD, Taylor D Jane (eds) Commentaries on research in breast diseases, vol 1. Liss, New York, pp 95–109

Nissen-Meyer R, Kjellgren K, Malmio K, Månsson B, Norin T (1978) Surgical adjuvant chemotherapy. Results with one short course with cyclophosphamide after mastectomy for breast cancer. Cancer 41: 2088–2098

Schabel FM (1977) Rationale for adjuvant chemotherapy. Cancer 39: 2875–2882

Appendix 1. Members of the Scandinavian Adjuvant Chemotherapy Study Group

In Finnland

Helsinki: AA. Järvinen †, L. Holsti, K. Malmio †
Oulu: G. Blanco, T. Larmi
Vasa: P.-O. Grönblom

In Norway

Akershus: T. Brøyn, N. Helsingen, F. W. Vaagenes
Bergen: L. Kolsaker, B. Rosengren, M. Tangen
Bodø : R. Capoferro, S. M. Sivertsen
Lillehammer: I. Hareide, S. K. Hjort
Oslo: I. O. Brennhovd, S. Gundersen, S. Hagen, T. Harbitz, H. Høst, O. G. Jørgensen, S. Kvaløy, H. O. Myhre, R. Nissen-Meyer (coordinator)

In Sweden

Borås: S. Ahlström, C.-A. Ekman, B. Månsson
Gävle: G. Hellström, T. Norin, G. Odén
Jönköping: I. Iacobaeus, B. Mårtensson
Kalmar: B. Pallin
Linköping: J. Sääf, D. Turesson
Norrköping: H. O. Ahnlund, K. Kjellgren, R. Peterhoff
Västervik: K. Wiegner

Preoperative Adjuvant Chemotherapy (Neoadjuvant) for Carcinoma of the Breast: Rationale and Safety Report

J. Ragaz, R. Baird, R. Rebbeck, A. Goldie, A. Coldman, and J. Spinelli

Cancer Control Agency of British Columbia,
2625 Healther Street, Vancouver, British Columbia V5Z 3J3, Canada

Introduction

The results of postoperative adjuvant chemotherapy for patients with high-risk carcinoma of the breast (Jones et al. 1981; Bonadonna et al. 1978) suggest an increase in disease-free survival compared with untreated controls. These results are by no means optimum. In the absence of new and more effective single chemotherapy agents for breast cancer, maximum effort should be made to explore the pharmacodynamics and scheduling of the standard chemotherapy regimens. Following this line of approach, we have started a programme that has led us in the past 2 years into the introduction of the study of preoperative adjuvant chemotherapy for breast cancer (Ragaz et al. 1981, 1982).

Rationale

Cancer occurs when one healthy cell undergoes mutation into one single cancer cell. It has been established that it will take as many as 30 doublings of the first malignant cell before the diagnosis can be made, by which time a size of 1–3 cm^3 will have been achieved. With only 12 more doublings a lethal tumour cell burden with the death of the host will be reached (Shackney and Ritch 1982). We can therefore see that at the time of diagnosis the tumour is usually advanced in its history, and the transition between the curative and palliative treatment is very narrow.

As the tumour grows in time, the increase of tumour cell burden per unit of time will decrease. In other words, later in the history of the tumour the proliferation rate of individual cells will decrease, and the doubling time of the tumour as an entity will increase. The observation that the more rapid exponential growth of the initial stages of the tumour will be replaced by exponential retardation in the later stages (expressed by the Gompertzian curve) has been confirmed by many investigators.

The reasons for the retarded growth of the aged tumour are multiple, but the most important result from the fact that in the more bulky tumours, a larger proportion of the cells is out of cycle, therefore not contributing directly to the growth. Because of the distance of the capillaries in more advanced tumours, a large part of the tumour is necrotic and some cells are removed from the area, or are eliminated by the defence mechanisms. In addition, some workers postulate production of chalone-like mechanisms by the tumour, which may cause a direct decrease of the proliferation rate and an increase in the doubling time (De Wys 1971).

Recent Results in Cancer Research. Vol. 98

These observations will make it easier to understand that a noncurative removal of the part of the tumour population – cytoreduction – will shift the proliferation rate of the remaining cells from the slow and flat portion of the Gompartzian curve into the steep part. There is good evidence from the experimental data available to suggest that noncurative cytoreduction – surgery (Simpson-Herren 1979. Gunduz and Fisher 1979), chemotherapy, and radiotherapy – decrease the doubling time of remaining cancer cells. It has also been suggested that in addition to the perturbation of the tumour, infection or stress can enhance the proliferation of the remaining cells (Saba 1978).

Can the subtle or sometimes more easily observed changes in tumour cell kinetics after noncurative surgery, well described in animal models, take place in human tumours? Anecdotal cases suggest that the answer is yes (El-Fiffi 1965. Lange et al. 1980). Well-documented reports, however, are not easily found in the literature.

We present here a case of a 53-year-old woman with breast cancer diagnosed in 1978, who developed a single 1-cm metastasis in the right lung in January 1980. The shadow grew slowly and the estimated doubling time between January 1980 and April 1981 was 80 days. In May 1981, both the whole-lung tomograms and the CAT scan of the lungs showed this to be a single 3- to 5-cm lesion. Subsequently, in late May 1981 the patient underwent thoracotomy and lobectomy, with resection of the lesion for curvative purpose. A chest x-ray taken 10 days after surgery showed no trace of malignancy. Two months later, however, on 11th August 1981, the patient presented with cough and fatigue, and the chest x-rays showed multiple bilateral lung metastases. This was followed by progressive onset of shortage of breath, a rapid downhill course despite treatment with chemotherapy and hormones, and an early death. Doubling time of the newly developed lesions after surgery was estimated at 25 days. We can say that in this particular patient, the noncurative surgery significantly changed the natural course of the previously documented metastatic lesion – a relatively slow-growing single lesion was replaced within days after surgery by rapidly growing multiple and bilateral metastases, proliferating significantly faster than the original lesion.

If the accelerated growth of established metastatic disease following noncurative surgery is a true phenomenon in advanced disease, it would be logical to postulate that the same biological effect can occur at the level of the nonmeasurable micrometastases following the removal of the primary tumour at the time of the mastectomy. If this is the case, then in the majority of stage II or III breast cancer patients (high likelihood of micrometastases present), the mastectomy itself can be viewed as an example of a noncurative surgery; thus the possibility exists that soon after surgery the remaining cancer cells may accelerate their division rate. In view of this theory, several animal studies on the protective effects of preoperative chemotherapy are of importance (Brock 1959; Corbett et al. 1981; Schabel 1979).

Corbett et al. (1981) have shown in an experiment with mice mammary tumours, that preoperative chemotherapy reduced the incidence of local recurrence and increased the life-span of the animals, compared with the controls treated by postoperative chemotherapy. Similarly, Schabel (1979) discussed a study of the same animal model (breast mammary tumour), in which preoperative treatment with adriamycin on day 12 followed by surgery on day 15 resulted in a significant prolongation of the life-span and improvement of the cure rate (63%) compared with the groups of animals treated by surgery on day 15 and adriamycin postoperatively on day 18 (cure rate 13%).

Schabel (1979) attributed the superior results of preoperative chemotherapy to the reduced tumour cell burden at the time of surgery owing to the institution of an early preoperative systemic treatment.

Using the Goldie and Coldman computer model (Goldie and Coldman 1979), we have simulated and calculated the percent probability (P%) of 5-year survival for patients receiving preoperative versus postoperative adjuvant chemotherapy. The model is based on the old concept of the Nobel Prize-winning work of Luria and Delbruk (1943) on the mutations of bacteria towards the resistance of infections with phage. It postulates that, similarly to bacteria, the malignant cells undergo spontaneous and continuous genetic mutations, and one of the phenotypic changes arising as a result of these mutations is an alteration of the state of responsiveness to the chemotherapy – the state of sensitivity to chemotherapy would be rapidly and spontaneously altered into the state of resistance to the same treatment. Although the concept is not new, the main contribution of the Goldie and Coldman model is the quantitative expression of the resistance to chemotherapy and the consideration in the mathematical calculation of the mutation rate – one of the most important factors determining the probability of having 0 or more than 0 resistant cells (state of 0 resistant cells = 100% probability of cure). One of the conclusions obtained with the model used in our work on preoperative adjuvant chemotherapy is the evidence that even a short delay in instituting the adjuvant chemotherapy can have an adverse effect on the benefit that it would otherwise have. Whether this postulate, so frequently found to be true in animal studies, will be confirmed in a clinical setting with breast cancer patients remains to be shown, but there are indications, as seen from the work of Nissen-Meyer, that it may be the case. In that Norwegian study (Nissen-Meyer 1979) it was shown that a delay of 2–4 weeks in instituting adjuvant chemotherapy in one hospital entirely abolished its beneficial effect, which had been documented in ten other hospitals in which patients received the adjuvant chemotherapy on day 1 after mastectomy.

The credibility of the Goldie-Coldman model increased after Skipper and his group in Alabama successfully matched the survival predictions of the model with the survival of large groups of animals treated with the same chemotherapy agents at different times in their tumour history (Skipper 1980). Using the model, we have calculated the percent probability (P%) of disease-free survival at 5-years for the patients treated with preoperative adjuvant chemotherapy on day −7 (7 days before mastectomy), and compared the P% with that of the patients treated with postoperative chemotherapy on day +28. For an estimated doubling time of 40 days (average doubling time for the human breast carcinoma tumour stem cells), the P% for preoperative chemotherapy on day −7 was 84%, whereas postoperative chemotherapy on day +28 resulted in P% of 73%. When, in addition to the delay of 35 days in instituting chemotherapy (difference between day −7 and day +28), we took into account a decrease in the doubling time of the tumour stem cells due to the suspected acceleration of their growth rate in connection with surgery, the P% for postoperative chemotherapy on day +28 was calculated at 70%, 64%, and 48% for tumours with estimated doubling times of 30, 20, and 10 days, respectively. This shows that the potential for cure may be decreased with a delay of 35 days in instituting treatment, and the P% will be inversely related to the doubling times. The higher probability of survival with preoperative than with postoperative treatment is directly related to the systemic tumour cell burden present at the time of initiation of chemotherapy. In the preoperative setting, the tumour cell burden was calculated as 4.3×10^4 cells (systemic micrometastases excluding the primary; (Skipper 1979) whereas the tumour cell burden at the time of postoperative chemotherapy on day +28 was calculated as 8.1×10^4 cells. Both calculations were based on tumours with fixed doubling times of 40 days. For the tumours with the simulated decrease of postsurgical doubling times of 30, 20, and 10 days, the tumour cell burden on day +28 after surgery was calculated as 9.5×10^4, 1.3×10^5, and 3.5×10^5 cells, respectively.

In conclusion, the model predicts a better outcome after treatment with an early preoperative chemotherapy than with a moderately delayed postoperative adjuvant chemotherapy given after the mastectomy.
The next concept in our work an preoperative adjuvant chemotherapy is the role of fine-needle aspiration (FNA) in obtaining the primary tissue diagnosis of breast cancer. Recently, FNA has received a great deal of attention in many centers in Europe and the United States of America, including our institute (Sager et al. 1980; Zajicek 1974; Rosen et al. 1972; Kern 1979; Salter and Bassett 1981; Pontifex and Suen 1981). It is a safe procedure, which can be performed immediately after a suggestive breast lump is diagnosed. The aspirate from the lump is obtained after application of suction by the syringe, and can be smeared on a glass, processed, and viewed with the Papanicolaou technique, the results being available within 30–60 minutes. In addition to the speed of the diagnosis – an important factor when an anxious woman, her family, and physicians are involved – it may be a safer procedure than the open biopsy, which is presently routinely performed in the majority of hospitals in North America. Open biopsy is quite commonly done as a separate procedure under a general anaesthetic, and the definitive surgery is then performed at a later date a few days afterwards. In light of the experimental data on adverse effects of surgery on the remaining malignant cells, open biopsy can indeed be regarded as an example of noncurative surgery. This may be the case as in many mastectomy specimens; there is a high yield of residual disease around the excisional biopsy. In addition, in the majority of stage II, III, and high-risk stage I patients, there is a high likelihood of systemic micrometastases. Because of the absence of general anaesthetic, tissue trauma, and tumour manipulation with FNA in comparison with open biopsy, one can postulate that FNA, in addition to being simpler and quicker, may indeed be a better procedure in relation to the tumour kinetics.
How accurate is FNA as the main diagnostic procedure for obtaining tissue diagnosis for breast carcinoma? Pooled results of 3,960 cases published in the literature (Sager et al. 1980, Zajicek 1974; Rosen et al. 1972) have shown that in the cases where carcinoma of the breast was subsequently well proven at the time of mastectomy, in 85% of the patients the condition was correctly diagnosed by FNA. False-negative results were obtained in 4.8% of patients, and 10.2% of the aspirates were nonsatisfactory on technical grounds, requiring subsequent confirmation by an open biopsy. In cases where definitive diagnosis was that of a benign tumour, the diagnosis with the help of FNA was correctly made in 80% of the cases. In 19.7% it was nonsatisfactory and 0.3% of the cases were false negative. If mammogram and clinical examinations were suggestive of carcinoma, a correct diagnosis by FNA was made in 99% of the cases. There were no instances of false-positive diagnosis, and diagnostic error was 1%. As a result of this development, many centres in Europe and North America are performing FNA with increasing frequency and the present consensus among researchers is that in experienced hands FNA could save a large number of patients an unnecessary hospitalization and the trauma of open biopsy (Salter and Bassett 1981; Pontifex and Suen 1981).

Study Design and Results

The pilot study of preoperative adjuvant chemotherapy at our institute started in January 1980. Because of the nature of the initial management of breast cancer, the surgeons associated with our institute played a pivotal role in the initial part of the programme. Besides establishing the tissue diagnosis of breast cancer, they were the first specialists to introduce to the patient and the family physician the subject of adjuvant chemotherapy and the entity of the preoperative adjuvant chemotherapy.

At the time of diagnosis, the patients were booked for definitive surgery in the same way as patients not receiving preoperative adjuvant chemotherapy. The adjuvant chemotherapy given before mastectomy consisted of cyclophosphamide, methotrexate, and 5-FU, given in the same way as in our regimen for adjuvant chemotherapy given after operation.

At the earliest possible time after a tissue diagnosis of breast carcinoma was obtained and after the initial investigations were ordered, patients were given their first course of adjuvant chemotherapy. The precise timing of the initiation of chemotherapy depended on the patient's willingness to participate in the study and on the surgeon's ability to organize the treatment. The analysis of our study has shown that the median interval between the day of diagnosis and the first day of adjuvant chemotherapy was 2.0 days (range 0–12, average 3.2 days). This is a substantial reduction from the mean delay of up to 35 days that is the average time interval between the diagnosis and initiation of adjuvant chemotherapy in most institutes in North America.

After surgery, the patients with positive axillary lymph nodes and those with negative axillary lymph nodes but with histological signs of high risk in the primary tumours (vascular invasion or lymphangitic spread) received a total of 6 months of adjuvant chemotherapy, with or without adjuvant radiotherapy in a similar fashion to our patients without preoperative chemotherapy. The axillary node-negative patients with low-risk tumours had no further chemotherapy after mastectomy.

Our analysis of the first 43 patients to receive one course of preoperative adjuvant chemotherapy has shown that one cycle of CMF preceding surgery by an average of 8 days was well tolerated. The time for mastectomy wound healing, the incidence of wound hematoma and infection, and the days an which postoperative fever, bone marrow and Gl toxicities, and other side-effects were recorded did not differ significantly from the corresponding data in patients receiving adjuvant chemotherapy postsurgically or undergoing mastectomy without preoperative adjuvant chemotherapy.

Conclusion

Indications are available from the literature to show that the old concept of breast cancer as an incurable disease may be slowly becoming outdated. The understanding of the nature and biology of breast cancer, in particular the recognition of its early systemic spread in the majority of the patients, the relatively high sensitivity of micrometastases to chemotherapy compared with the treatment of metastatic disease, and increasing knowledge of the pharmacological principles of combination chemotherapy and tumour kinetics have led oncologists to introduce early adjuvant chemotherapy trials in the last two decades. Despite the frequent minor or major disappointments with this treatment, there is a steadily growing consensus that a correctly administered combination of systemic and local therapies is showing a beneficial impact on the survival of patients with breast cancer.

Our concept and rationale for preoperative adjuvant chemotherapy links the advances in adjuvant therapies in general with the principles of the Goldie-Coldman model with its stress on the importance of the timing of the adjuvant chemotherapy. It also takes into consideration the observations on tumour cell kinetics, in particular the suspected acceleration of the proliferation rate of the remaining cancer cells after the noncurative surgery.

Can early preoperative chemotherapy prevent the increased proliferation of the micrometastases? The answer is not clear, but it is suspected that like radiation, chemotherapy will have two effects: (a) It will effectively eradicate and kill the most sensitive cells; and (b) it will generate a population of "doomed" cells, which may go through one or more cell division cycles but will die soon afterwards. In both instances it will effectively reduce the quantity of the local and systemic clonogenic tumour cells, which are at high risk for decreasing their doubling time in connection with the surgery, as well as increasing their resistance to the chemotherapy soon afterwards. Preoperative adjuvant chemotherapy would treat the tumour at the earliest possible time in its history after the diagnosis has been made, thus maximally decreasing the chance of having to deal with spontaneously occurring resistant mutants. In addition, an effective reduction of the size of the primary tumour and its surrounding micrometastases may improve the quality of the mastectomy and decrease the incidence of local recurrence.

Reviewing the literature and experimental data, we are suggesting that the rationale for an early preoperative adjuvant chemotherapy is very logical and sound, and does deserve further investigations. Furthermore, we conclude from our pilot study of the first 43 patients treated with preoperative adjuvant chemotherapy that one course of adjuvant CMF chemotherapy several days before mastectomy is safe.

We are presently starting a randomized study of preoperative versus postoperative adjuvant chemotherapy to document whether the new approach to the timing of chemotherapy in relation to mastectomy will have any impact on the total survival.

References

Bonadonna G, Valagussa P, Rossi A (1978) Are surgical adjuvant trials altering the course of breast cancer? Semin Oncol 5: 450

Brock N (1959) Neue experimentelle Ergebnisse mit N-Lost-Phosphamidestern. Strahlentherapie

Corbett TH, Griswold DP, Roberts JB, Schabel FM (1981) Cytotoxic adjuvant therapy and the experimental model. In: Stoll BA (ed) Systemic control of breast cancer. Heinemann, London pp 204–243

De Wys WD (1972) Studies correlating the growth rate of a tumour and its metastases and providing evidence for tumour related systemic growth retarding factors. Cancer Res 32: 324–379

El-Fiffi (1965) Increased incidence of pulmonary metastases after celiotomy. Arch Surg 91: 625

Goldie JH, Coldman AJ (1979) A methematical model for relating the drug sensitivity of tumour to their spontaneous mutation rate. Cancer Treat Rep 63: 1717–1733

Gunduz N, Fisher B (1979) Effect of surgical removal of the growth and kinetics of residual tumour. Caner Res 39: 3861–3865

Jones S, Moon T, Davis S (1981) Comparative analysis of selected breast Ca adjuvant trials in relation to the natural history data base (NHBD). In: Salmon SE, Jones SE (eds) Adjuvant therapy of cancer, vol III. Grune and Stratton, New York, pp 483–491

Kern WH (1979) Diagnosis of breast cancer by fine needle aspiration smears. JAMA 11: 241

Lange PH, Hekmat K, Bosl G, Kennedy BJ, Fraley EE (1980) Accelerated growth of testicular cancer after cytoreductive surgery. Cancer 45: 1498–1506

Luria SE, Delbruck M (1943) Mutations of bacteria from viral sensitivity to viral resistance. Genetics 28: 4921

Nissen-Meyer R (1979) One short chemotherapy course in primary breast cancer: 12 year followup series I of the Scandinavian Adjuvant Chemotherapy Study Group. In: Salmon SE, Jones SE (eds) Adjuvant therapy of cancer II. Grune and Stratton, New York, pp 207–217

Pontifex AH, Suen KC (1981) Fine needle aspiration diagnosis of breast masses. Br Cancer Med J 23: 542–543

Ragaz J, Baird R, Rebbeck P (1981) Preoperative chemotherapy for Ca of the breast – safety report. Third International Conference on Adjuvant Therapy of Cancer, 18–21 March, Tucson, Ariz. (abstr. no 9)

Ragaz J, Goldie JH, Coldman A (1982) Preoperative adjuvant chemotherapy for Ca of the breast. Am Soc Clin Oncol 1: 87 (C-337, abstr)

Rosen R, Hajdu SI, Robins G (1972) Diagnosis of carcinoma of the breast by aspiration biopsy. Surg Gynecol Obstet 134: 837–838

Saba TM (1978) Prevention of liver endothelial systemic host defence failure after surgery by intravenous opsonic glycoprotein therapy. Ann Surg 188: 142–152

Sager GF, Taxiarchis LM, Bowdoin BH (1980) Fine needle aspiration breast biopsy. A 6 year experience with 1,034 aspirations. JAMA 71: 49–59

Salter DR, Bassett AA (1981) Role of needle aspiration in reducing the number of unnecessary breast biopsies. J Surg 24: 311–313

Schabel FM (1979) Recent studies with surgical adjuvant chemotherapy or immunotherapy of metastatic solid tumours. In: Jones SE (ed) Adjuvant therapy of cancer, vol II. Grune and Stratton, New York

Shackney SS, Ritch PS, Cell kinetics. In: Chabner B (ed) Pharmacological principles of cancer treatment. Saunders, Toronto

Simpson-Herren L (1979) Effects of surgery on the cell kinetics of residual tumour. Cancer Treat Rep 63: 1717–1733

Skipper HE (1979) Repopulation rates of breast cancer after mastectomy (judged from breakpoint in remission duration curves). University Microfilm International, Ann Arbo

Skipper HE (1980) Some thoughts regarding a recent publication. In: Goldie JH, Coldman AJ (eds) A mathematical model for relating the drug sensitivity of tumour to their spontaneous mutation rate. University Microfilm International, Ann Arbor

Zajicek J (1974) Aspiration biopsy cytology, part 1: Cytology of supra diaphragmatic organs. Karger, New York (Monographs in clinical cytology)

Perioperative and Conventionally Timed Chemotherapy in Operable Breast Cancer

A. Goldhirsch*

Ludwig Institut für Krebsforschung, Inselspital,
3010 Bern, Switzerland

Introduction

Adjuvant chemotherapy with CMF in pathological stage II breast cancer has been shown by the Milan Group to produce a disease-free survival and overall survival advantage at 6 years in premenopausal patients (Bonadonna et al. 1978). The value of adjuvant chemotherapy in postmenopausal patients is less well established, although it seems likely to be real. It has been suggested that treatment success may well be dose related in all patients (Bonadonna and Valagussa 1981) and toxicity related (Carpenter et al. 1982). The role of adjuvant chemotherapy in node-negative patients has still to be confirmed (Senn et al. 1981).

A number of strategies have been proposed in recent years to improve on results of current adjuvant therapy. These include:

1. Non-cross-resistant combination of drugs.
2. More intensive and prolonged use of existing drugs.
3. Investigational drugs.
4. Combination of chemo- and hormonotherapy and/or immunotherapy
5. Early commencement of chemotherapy after surgery.

Sequential use of non-cross-resistant drugs and more intensive chemotherapy are being evaluated by other groups. The current group of investigational drugs seems unlikely to be better, in the adjuvant context, than existing ones.

The Ludwig Breast Cancer Studies I–IV have explored chemo-/hormonotherapy combinations during the past years, and additional follow-up is warranted to make significant data available from these trials.

Based upon experimental, kinetic and drug resistance considerations (Goldie and Coldman 1979; Schabel 1977; DeWys 1972) and some clinical evidence (Fisher et al. 1975; Nissen-Meyer et al. 1978), it has been suggested that the time of starting chemotherapy after removal of the primary tumor may be of critical importance.

In fact, two clinical trials in which chemotherapy was started in the immediate postoperative period showed survival advantages in at least some of the patients treated. The NSABP study using perioperative thio-TEPA produced a significant survival advantage in premenopausal patients with four or more nodes involved (Fisher et al.

* For the Ludwig Breast Cancer Study Group; list of participants in Appendix 1

Recent Results in Cancer Research. Vol. 98

1975). The Scandinavian Adjuvant Chemotherapy Group Study (Nissen-Meyer et al. 1978) used cyclophosphamide and found a survival advantage of 11% overall after 12 years. This benefit applied almost equally to N(+) and N(−), pre- and postmenopausal patients and was lost when this therapy was delayed by as little as 3 weeks. It seems therefore rational, even essential, to evaluate the effects of starting chemotherapy immediately after surgery rather than exposing the patient to the possible deleterious effect of delay.

Study Design

To study this aspect of timing in the adjuvant treatment of breast cancer the Ludwig Breast Cancer Study Group started a trial using a perioperative treatment given in the immediate postoperative phase. The study design is reported in Fig. 1.

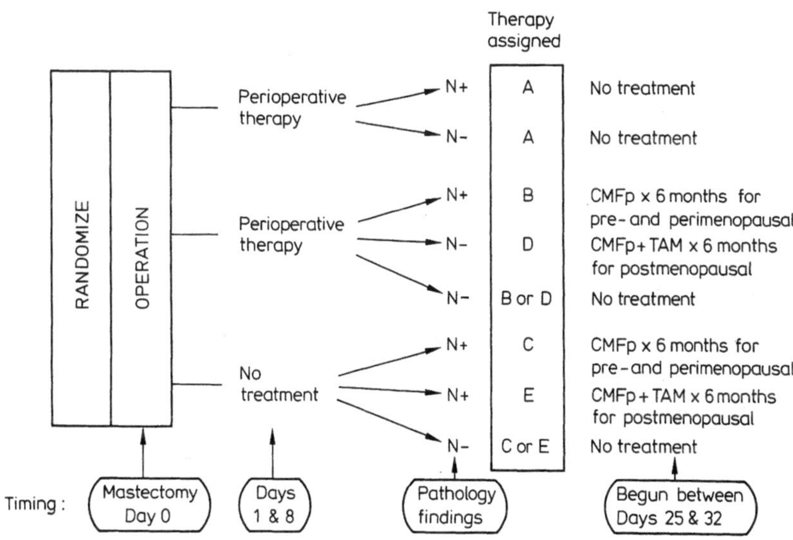

Perioperative therapy: (Begin within 36 h after mastectomy)

Cyclophosphamide	– 400 mg/m² IV	Days 1 & 8
Methotrexate	– 40 mg/m² IV	
5-Fluorouracil	– 600 mg/m² IV	
*Leucovorin	15 mg IV 24 h after day 1 and 15 mg IV 24 h after day 8	

Conventionally timed adjuvant therapy: (Begins 25–32 days after mastectomy)

Cyclophosphamide	– 100 mg/m²PO	days 1–14	Every 28 Days
Methotrexate	– 40 mg/m²IV	days 1 & 8	
5-Fluorouracil	– 600 mg/m²IV	days 1 & 8	
Prednisone	– 7.5 mg/m PO	daily	
Tamoxifen	– 20 mg PO	daily	

Fig. 1. Schematic showing design of the Ludwig Breast Cancer Study V. * Leucovorin was added after 12 months

It should be stressed that two-thirds of the node-negative patients receive perioperative chemotherapy only, while one-third receive no further therapy after the mastectomy. For the N+ patients, one-third receive only conventionally timed chemotherapy starting within 25–36 days after mastectomy, one-third receive only the perioperative chemotherapy, and one-third receive both perioperative chemotherapy and conventionally timed chemotherapy.

Trial Logistics

Assigned perioperative therapy must commence within 36 hours of mastectomy. Thus, it was necessary to evolve a satisfactory system for rapid central registration and randomization (Gelber, this volume). Randomization can be done immediately after mastectomy to allow chemotherapy to be given on the first postoperative day, or prior to mastectomy and before a histological diagnosis has been obtained. If the patient's breast lesion were found to be histologically benign, then trial entry would be cancelled. Because of time zone differences, randomization must be carried out in Bern, Switzerland and in Sydney, Australia. Stratification is by clinical and menopausal status. The definition of menopausal status is described in Table 1.

Surgery

Total mastectomy with complete axillary clearance is the standard surgical procedure. This is carried out with or without removal of the pectoralis muscle(s). The important requirements of the protocol are: All breast tissue must be removed; a minimum of eight axillary lymph nodes must be available for histological examination; a specimen must be prepared for estrogen receptor assay.

Table 1. Menopausal Status

Premenopausal and Perimenopausal	Age > 52 years and LNMP (last normal menstrual period) within 1 year, *or* Age ≤ 52 years of and LNMP within 3 years, or menstruating, *or* Age ≤ 55 years and hysterectomy but no bilateral oophorectomy, *or* Biochemical confirmation of continuing ovarian function (for doubtful patients)
Postmenopausal	Age > 52 years with 1 years of amenorrhea, *or* Age ≤ 52 years with 3 years of amenorrhea or more, *or* Age > 55 and history of hysterectomy without bilateral oophorectomy *or* Biochemical evidence of cessation of ovarian function (for doubtful patients)

Eligibility Criteria

These include histologically confirmed breast cancer, preoperative leukocyte count $\geq 4{,}000/mm^3$, platelet count $\geq 100{,}000/mm^3$, serum creatinine ≤ 1.5 mg%, or < 130 μmol/l, bilirubin ≤ 1.5 mg% or ≤ 20μmol/l, SGOT ≤ 60 IU/l, and UICC performance status 0–2 preoperatively. Patients with prior therapy for breast cancer, other malignant disease, biopsy in a period of more than 21 days prior to mastectomy, and surgical risks are ineligible for entry on study.

Perioperative Chemotherapy (Immediately After Surgery = PeCT)

The combinations including cyclophosphamide (C), methotrexate (M), and 5-fluorouracil (F) are the most widely used and evaluated regimens as adjuvant cytotoxic treatment to surgery in breast cancer. They were therefore a logical choice for perioperative use in this study. The regimen includes: C 400 mg/m^2 IV; M 40 mg/m^2 IV; and F = 600 mg/m^2 IV on days 1 and 8. The IV route was chosen to insure delivery and ease administration in patients who have just undergone surgery. PeCT should be delivered within 36 hours after completion of mastectomy.

A pilot study of 65 patients treated with this regimen indicated that tolerance was acceptable. However, since initiation of the randomized trial, unacceptable and unpredictable toxicity has been observed during the first year of patient accrual. The evaluation of the postoperative course after the administration of the PeCT showed a correlation between the occurrence of severe or potentially severe complications and some factors related to the patient and to the chemotherapy schedule. Factors related to the patient were found to be age and renal function. Factors related to the chemotherapy schedule were found to be time from mastectomy to chemotherapy administration and the dose given on day 1. Because of the possibility that toxicity reflected an interaction between methotrexate and nitrous oxide anesthesia (Nunn et al. 1982; Deacon et al. 1980; Kono et al. 1981), folinic acid rescue was added 24 hours after days 1 (IV) and 8 (PO) of the perioperative cycle (Dudman et al. 1982). Furthermore, patients 66 years of age or older were excluded from the trial. Requirements for close monitoring of the patient in the postoperative phase were included. An evaluation and report of this toxicity will be presented soon (Ludwig Breast Cancer Study Group, to be published).

Conventionally Timed Adjuvant Therapy (Con. CT)

The justification for using CMF is largely historical. Low-dose prednisone was included because of the Group's own data showing that higher cytotoxic doses are tolerated with this agent. Tamoxifen was included in the postmenopausal regimen because of the higher response rate in conjunction with combination chemotherapy in advanced disease and because of some positive results in ongoing adjuvant trials (Hubay et al. 1980; Fisher et al. 1981). The 6-month duration of this "portion" of adjuvant treatment is based upon current reports from Milan and Switzerland (Bonadonna et al. 1981; Jungi et al. 1981).

Dose Modification of Chemotherapy

Full doses of cytotoxic drugs are given in the absence of neurotoxicity, mucosal toxicity, and infection. Normal renal and hepatic functions are necessary for the full dose delivery. A dose reduction is undertaken if white blood cell and platelet counts indicate mild myelosuppression. As reported previously, special requirements for the treatment and follow-up of patients in the immediately postoperative phase were included. Close monitoring of the patient, especially the hematological and renal toxicities, was added as a further requirement. Intravenous fluids were added during the first 36 hours postoperatively. Investigators were alerted to the onset of stomatitis, diarrhea, and early blood cell counts falling within 2 or 3 days after drug administration as premonitory signs for severe MTX toxicity.

Pathology Central Review

The pathology central review laboratory has been set up for evaluation of the diagnosis, classification, and grading of the primary tumor, the nontumor breast tissue, and local or regional spread found in the biopsy and/or mastectomy specimen, including the axillary lymph nodes. All grossly negative lymph nodes are examined microscopically. A minimum of at least eight axillary lymph nodes are examined from each patient. Determination of treatment is based upon the evaluation of lymph node involvement by the responsible pathologist of the participating institution.

Hormone Receptor Determination

Determination of estrogen receptor and progesterone receptor status in the tumor tissue is standardized and quality controlled on a group scale.

Table 2. Patient accrual (November 1981 to December 1982) in the Ludwig Breast Cancer Study V

Institution	No of patients
Auckland	33
Cape Town	49
Essen/Düsseldorf	49
Gothenburg	194
Ljubljana (late entry)	17
Madrid	67
Melbourne	77
Perth	38
Sydney	38
Swiss Group (SAKK)	170
	732

Patient Accrual

Patient accrual was started in November 1981 and entry as of January 1983 is presented in Table 2. It is necessary to have 550 patients with axillary node involvement for each treatment arm to insure the statistical validity of the results (Gelber, this volume). The revised program with leucovorin rescue has been in effect for the past 3 months. An evaluation of the toxicity observed for the modified regimen will be conducted when a comparable number of patients are available for analysis.

Appendix 1. Ludwig Breast cancer study group

Institution	Investigators
Ludwig Institute for Cancer Research, Inselspital, Bern, Switzerland	A. Goldhirsch (*Study Coordinator*), W. Hartmann, B. Davis, R. Bettelheim (*Study Pathologists*), D. Zava, C. Ramminger, C. Wiedmer
Harvard School of Public Health and Dana-Farber Cancer Center, Boston, U.S.A.	R. Gelber (*Study Statistician*), K. Price, M. Zelen
Frontier Science & Tech. Res. Found., Buffalo, U.S.A.	M. Isley, M. Parsons, L. Szymoniak
Auckland Breast Cancer Study Group, Auckland, New Zealand	R. G. Kay, J. Probert, B. Mason, H. Wood, E. G. Gifford, J. F. Carter, J. C. Gillmann, J. Anderson, L. Yee, I. M. Holdaway, G. C. Hitchcock, M. Jagusch
Groote Schuur Hospital, Cape Twon, Rep. of South Africa	A. Hacking, D. M. Dent, J. Terblanche, A. Tilmann A. Gudgeon, E. Dowdle, R. Sealy, P. Palmer
Spedali Civili & Fondazione Beretta, Brescia, Italy	G. Marini, E. Simoncini, P. Marpicati, U. Sartori, A. Barni, L. Morassi, P. Grigolato, D. Di Lorenzo, A. Albertini, G. Marinone, M. Zorzi
University of Essen, West German Tumor Center, Essen, University of Düsseldorf, West-Germany	C. G. Schmidt, F. Schüning, K. Höffken, L. D. Leder, H. Ludwig, R. Callies, P. Faber, H. G. Schnürch, H. H. Bender, H. Bojar
Swedish Western Breast Cancer Study Group, Göteborg, Sweden	C.-M. Rudenstam, E. Cahlin, H. Salander, I. Branehög, G. Jäderström, R. Hultborn, U. Wannholt, S. Nilsson, J. Fornander, J. Säve-Söderbergh, CH. Johnsén, O. Ruusvik, G. Ostberg, L. Mattson, C. G. Bäckström, S. Bergegardh. U. Ljungqvist, I. Dahl, Y. Hessman, S. Holmberg, S. Dahlin, G. Wallin
The Institute Oncology, Ljubljana, Yugoslavia	J. Lindtner, J. Novak, J. Cervek, O. Cerar, P. Mavec, R. Golouh, J. Lamovec, J. Jancar, S. Sebek
Madrid Breast Cancer Group, Madrid, Spain	H. Cortés-Funes, F. Martinez-Tello, F. Cruz Caro, M. L. Marcos, M. A. Figueras, F. Calero, A. Suarez, F. Pastrana, R. Huertas
Anti-Cancer Council of Victoria, Melbourne, Australia	J. Collins, R. Snyder, R. Bennett, J. Burns, J. F. Forbes, J. Funder, E. Guli, L. Harrison, S. Hart, P. Kitchen, R. Lovell, R. Reed, I. Russel, A. Shaw, L. Sisely, R. D. Snyder, P. Jeal, J. M. Colebatch
Sir Charles Gairdner Hospital Nedlands, Western Australia	M. Byrne, P. M. Reynolds, H. J. Sheiner, S. Levitt, D. Kernmode, K. B. Shilkin, R. Hähnel

Appendix 1. (continued)

Institution	Investigators
SAKK (Swiss Group for Clin. Cancer Res.)	
– Bern, Inselspital	K. Brunner, P. Aeberhard, H. Cottier, K. Burki, A. Zimmermann, E. Dreher, G. Locher, M. Berger, M. Walther, R. Joss, A. Gervasi, M. Castiglione, U. Herrmann, P. Herrmann
– St. Gallen, Kantonsspital	W. F. Jungi, H. J. Senn, A. Mutzner, U. Schmid, Th. Hardmeier, E. Hochuli, O. Schildknecht
– Bellinzona, Ospedale San Giovanni	F. Cavalli, M. Varini, P. Luscieti, E. S. Passega, G. Losa
– Basel, Kantonsspital	J. P. Obrecht, F. Harder, A. C. Almendral, U. Eppenberger, J. Torhorst
– Geneva, Hôpital Cantonal Universitaire	P. Alberto, F. Krauer, R. Egeli, R. Mégevand, M. Forni, P. Schäfer, E. Jacot des Combes, A. M. Schindler, F. Misset
– Lausanne, CHUV	S. Leyvraz
– Neuchâtel, Hôpital des Cadolles	P. Siegenthaler, V. Barrelet, R. P. Baumann
– Luzern, Kantonsspital	H. J. Schmid
Ludwig Institute for Cancer Research, and Royal Prince Alfred Hospital, Sydney, Australia	M. H. N. Tattersall, R. Fox, A. Coates, D. Hedley, D. Raghavan, F. Niesche, R. West, S. Renwick, D. Green, J. Donovan, P. Duval, A. Ng, T. Foo, D. Glenn, T. J. Nash, R. A. North, J. Beith, G. O'Connor
Wellington Hospital, Wellington, New Zealand	J. S. Simpson, L. Hollaway, C. Unsworth

References

Bonadonna G, Valagussa P (1981) Dose-response effect of adjuvant chemotherapy in breast cancer. N Engl J Med 304: 20–51

Bonadonna G, Valagussa P, Rossi A, Zucali R, Tancini G, Bajetta E, Brambilla C, De Lena M, Di Fronzo G, Banfi A, Rilke F, Veronesi U (1978) Are surgical adjuvant trials altering the course of breast cancer? Semin Oncol 5: 450–464

Bonadonna G, Rossi A, Tancini G, Brambilla C, Marchini S, Valagussa P, Veronesi U (1981) Adjuvant treatment for breast cancer. The Milan Institute experience. Proceed was of the 3rd international conference on the adjuvant therapy of cancer. March 18–21, Tucson

Carpenter TT, Maddox WA, Laws HL, Wirtschaften DD, Soong SJ (1982) Favorable factors in the adjuvant therapy of breast cancer. Cancer 50: 18–23

Deacon R, Lumb M, Perry J (1980) Inactivation of methionine syntetase by nitrous oxide. Eur J Biochem 104: 419–422

DeWys WD (1972) Studies correlating the growth rate of a tumor and its metastases and providing evidence for tumor-related systemic growth-retarding factors. Cancer Res 32:374–379

Dudman NPB, Slowiaczek P, Tattersall MHN (1982) Methotrexate rescue by 5-methyl THF or 5-formyl THF in lymphoblastoid cell lines. Cancer Res 42:502–507

Fisher B, Slack N, Katrych D, Wolmark N (1975) Ten year follow-up of patients with carcinoma of the breast in a cooperative clinical trial evaluating surgical adjuvant chemotherapy. Surg Gynecol Obstet 140:528–534

Fisher B, Redmond C, Brown A, Wickerham DL, Wolmark N, Allegra J, Fischer G, Lippman M, Savlov E, Wittliff J, Fischer ER (1981) Treatment of primary breast cancer with chemotherapy and tamoxifen. N Engl J Med 305: 1–6

Goldie JH, Coldman AJ (1979) A mathematic model of relating the drug sensitivity of tumors to their spontaneous mutation rate. Cancer Treat Rep 63: 1727–1733

Hubay CA, Pearson OH, Marshall JS, Stellato TA, Rhodes RS, Be Banne SM (1980) Antiestrogen, cytotoxic chemotherapy and bacillus Calmette-Guerin vaccination in stage II breast cancer; a preliminary report. Surgery 87: 494–501

Jungi WF, Brunner KW, Cavalli F, Martz G, Rosset G, Barrelet L (1981) Short or long term adjuvant chemotherapy for breast cancer. Proc Am Soc Clin Oncol 22: 435 (Abstract C399)

Kano Y, Sakamoto S, Sakuraya K, Kuboto T, Hida K, Suda K, Takaku F (1981) Effect of nitrous oxide on human bone marrow cells and its synergistic effect with methionine and methotrexate on functional folate deficiency. Cancer Res 41: 4698–4701

Ludwig Breast Cancer Study Group (1983) Severe toxicity encountered in adjuvant combination chemotherapy for breast cancer administered in the immediate post-mastectomy period. Lancet II: 542–544

Nissen-Meyer R, Kjellgren K, Malmio K, Mansson B, Norin T (1978) Surgical adjuvant chemotherapy. Results with one short course with cyclophosphamide after mastectomy for breast cancer. Cancer 41: 2088–2098

Nunn JF, Sharer NM, Gorchein A, Jones JA, Wickramasingha SN (1982) Megaloblastic haemopoiesis after multiple short term exposure to nitrous oxide. Lancet I: 1379–1381

Schabel FM (1977) Surgical adjuvant chemotherapy of metastatic murine tumors. Cancer 40: 558–568

Senn HJ, Jungi WF, Amgwerd R (1981) Chemoimmunotherapy with LMF plus BCG in node-positive and node-positive breast cancer. In: Adjuvant therapy for cancer III. Salmon SE, Jones SE (eds). Grune and Stratton, New York, 385–390

Panel Discussion: Perioperative Chemotherapy for Breast Cancer

Moderated by K. W. Brunner (Bern), the second panel discussion dealt with perioperative chemotherapy in breast cancer. Preoperative chemotherapy as presented extensively by the Hellenic Breast Cooperative Group may have some potential for advanced stage III disease and there are certainly some interesting aspects (chemosensitivity testing in vivo, tumor shrinkage, immunostimulation?) to this approach, but it has clearly been felt that this type of chemotherapy so far has no proven clinical evidence of advantage in less advanced disease where preoperative chemotherapy might preclude some patients from potentially curative surgery. This is in contrast to osteosarcoma (see below) and many childhood solid tumors, and is possibly due to factors such as chemosensitivity and tumor growth. True perioperative chemotherapy, as reported by R. Nissen-Meyer and the Scandinavian Adjuvant Chemotherapy Study Group, resulted in a significantly prolonged relapse-free survival. Interestingly, the benefit was found both in stage I and in stage II, and in premenopausal as well as in postmenopausal patients. Compared with many other adjuvant trials showing widely differing degrees of benefit among the patient subgroups, the results in the first Scandinavian study uniformly support immediate postoperative chemotherapy, possibly indicating a different mechanism of action. More interestingly, preliminary analysis of the second study shows the old single-drug cyclophosphamide therapy to be at least as effective as the conventionally timed CMF multidrug regimen. This again could indicate that perioperative chemotherapy has different mechanisms of action than conventionally timed adjuvant therapy given 3 or even more weeks after surgery. Chemotherapy added at the time of surgery is more likely to take advantage of the altered cell kinetic of remaining micrometastases following removal of the primary tumor, and perioperative chemotherapy may better control tumor cells shed into the circulation during surgery.

Based on the mathematical model of Goldie and Coldman – the quantitative expression of resistance to chemotherapy by calculation of the mutation rate from sensitive to resistant cells (state of 0 resistant cells = 100% probability of cure) – theoretically chemotherapy should be given as soon as the diagnosis of cancer is established, immediately after positive tissue biopsy. However, the state of 0 resistant cells is very unlikely even in early clinical stages, since these small palpable lesions are already composed of 10^8 to 10^9 tumor cells with a considerable chance of cure by surgery alone. On the other hand, it is not known whether the mutation rate is influenced by the surgical reduction of tumor cells to the 10^2 or 10^3 level.

Probably the most appropriate clinical multicenter study evaluating perioperative chemotherapy in breast cancer is the currently ongoing Ludwig V Study presented by

A. Goldhirsch. This well-designed and well-documented trial raised the question of the maximum tolerated level of toxicity in perioperative chemotherapy. It was unanimously stated that there should be no deaths attributable to chemotherapy in potentially cured patients, since precise pathological staging is not available at the start of adjuvant treatment. Since protocol modification no more fatalities have been registered in the Ludwig trial. Two of the three toxic deaths reported among the first 360 evaluable patients were due at least in part to the lack of experience in this type of adjuvant chemotherapy, indicating the absolute necessity for close cooperation between medical oncologists and cancer surgeons.

Routine use of prophylactic antibiotics was not generally recommended for breast cancer patients receiving perioperative chemotherapy. It was concluded that antibiotic prophylaxis should be given according to the standard surgical rules irrespective of whether the patient will receive perioperative chemotherapy or not. It has been estimated that the most critical period for infectious complications is day 3–6 after surgery, whereas perioperative chemotherapy in currently ongoing trials is usually administered on days 1 and 8 after surgery. Much more clinical experience is needed to analyze the possible interferences of anesthesia and perioperative chemotherapy drugs, e.g., pulmonary toxicity of bleomycin, altered folate metabolism by nitrous oxide anesthesia. Our current knowledge of perioperative chemotherapy in breast cancer has been best characterized by R. Nissen-Meyer: "We need many large trials to answer all questions concerning type, timing, dosage, and combination of adjuvant chemotherapy agents in the perioperative setting."

Perioperative and Adjuvant Chemotherapy in Gastric Cancer

P. Schlag and W. Schreml

Sektion Chirurgische Onkologie, Chirurgische Universitätsklinik
Im Neuenheimer Feld 110, 6900 Heidelberg, Germany

Introduction

In spite of the more extensive and standardized surgical procedure now used, there have so far been only minor changes in the therapeutic results obtained in gastric cancer (Herfarth and Schlag 1979). In view of this, no further improvement of prognosis can be expected from the surgical approach only. This situation demands other therapeutic modalities that could improve the therapeutic results in this disease. One approach consists in perioperative chemotherapy, which can be administered before, during, or after the surgical intervention. The results that have been achieved with this regimen are reviewed below.

Postoperative Short-Term Single-Agent Chemotherapy

In the first trial of perioperative chemotherapy in gastric cancer the cytostatic agent thio-TEPA was administered either IP or IV, with the intention of killing tumor cells that had been seeded out during the operative procedure (Dixon et al. 1971; Longmire et al. 1968). This study by the Veterans Administration Surgical Oncology Group showed no improvement in survival time (Table 1). With this regimen there was even evidence of a deterioration in prognosis for a subset of patients who had undergone splenectomy during the gastric resection (Dixon et al. 1971). The VA Surgical Adjuvant Group next ran a study using fluorodesoxyuridin as the anticancer drug (Dwight et al. 1973; Serlin et al. 1969). Randomization was carried out on the first postoperative day and those patients selected to

Table 1. Controlled trials of perioperative chemotherapy following curative resection for gastric cancer: Postoperative short-term single-agent chemotherapy

Group	Number of patients	Drug	Survival benefit for treated patients
VASOG (1965)	194	Thio-TEPA	No improvement
VASOG (1969)	276	FUDR	No improvement
Imanage and Nakazato (1977)	669	Mitomycin C	Significant improvement

receive the drug were given an IV dose on each of days 1, 2, and 3 after the operation. The second course was then instituted between the 35th and 45th postoperative days. Analysis of the survival data in this study also showed no demonstrable benefit of treatment. Whether the failure should be attributed to the treatment plan or to the in our present view poor effect of the cytostatic drugs remains an open question.

Preoperative Chemotherapy

The very small and few studies with preoperative, especially intra-arterial, single-agent chemotherapy do not allow valid conclusions (Table 2). The approaches so far undertaken have not been satisfactory and the results are fairly negative (Fujimoto et al. 1976; Jinnai and Higashi 1976).

Postoperative Long-Term Single-Agent Chemotherapy

The results have led other groups to concentrate more on long-term postoperative chemotherapy. This therapeutic modality not only focuses on killing tumor cells that have been distributed systemically by the operative procedure but at the same time aims at the elimination of possible metastases. The above treatment concept has been defined as adjuvant chemotherapy (Burchenal 1976). The numerous studies that have been undertaken under this premise reflect a general approach of transferring therapies that are active in advanced disease into the minimal residual disease setting, in an attempt to prevent or delay recurrence (Table 3). Historically, the significance of the single agents 5-FU and mitomycin C as adjuvant treatment was first tested. Using mitomycin C, Imanaga reported an increase in survival especially for patients with stage II carcinomas (Imanaga and Nakazato 1977). Fujimoto et al. (1977) improved prognosis in a group of patients with gastric cancer by long-term chemotherapy with fluoropyrimidines. Whereas in this study patients who had tumor infiltration of the serosa showed improvement, the trial of Imanaga gave better results for patients without serosa invasion. It has not yet been possible to reproduce these results in other investigations (Hattori et al. 1972; Koyama 1978; Schlag et al. 1979). Therefore, these positive findings should be regarded with some reservation. It can thus be stated that intra- or postoperative monochemotherapy is of no certain value for the survival time of patients undergoing potentially curative gastric resection.

Table 2. Controlled trials of perioperative chemotherapy following curative resection for gastric cancer: Preoperative chemotherapy

Group	Number of patients	Drug(s)	Survival benefit for treated patients
Jinnai and Higashi (1976)	297	Mitomycin C	„Particularly beneficial“
Fujimoto et al. (1976)	62	5–FU Mitomycin C MTX	Not conclusive

Table 3. Controlled trials of perioperative chemotherapy following curative resection for gastric cancer: Postoperative long-term polychemotherapy

Group	Number of patients	Drug	Survival benefit for treated patients
VASOG (1982)	275	5-FU + methyl-CCNU	No improvement
GITSG (1982)	142	5-FU + methyl-CCNU	Significant improvement
Schlag et al. Own study (1982)	103	5-FU + BCNU	No improvement
Blake et al. (1981)	63	CMFV	No improvement
SWOG	–	FAM	In progress
EORTC	–	FAM	In progress

Table 4. Controlled trials of perioperative chemotherapy following curative resection for gastric cancer: Postoperative radio-chemotherapy

Group	Number of patients	Drug and radiation dose	Survival benefit for treated patients
EORTC (1981)	98	5-FU (short or longterm) + 55 Gy	Not conclusive
Dent et al. (1979)	142	5-FU + 20 Gy	No improvement
Mayo Clinic		5-FU + 30 Gy	In progress

Postoperative Radio-/Chemotherapy

In view of the experience with perioperative chemotherapy the question has been raised as to whether intra- or postoperative systemic chemotherapy is likely to reduce the local relapse rate, in particular, which is the major factor limiting therapeutic success in gastric cancer (Herfarth and Schlag 1979). A combined chemo- and radiotherapeutic approach seemed a promising idea (Table 4), but has not proved significantly effective in trials so far (Dent et al. 1979; Goffin et al. 1978).

Postoperative Long-Term Polychemotherapy

Since for metastatic gastric cancer combination chemotherapy has proved to be superior over single-agent cytostatic therapy, it was presumed that the combinations would also be more active in the surgical adjuvant situation. One possibility is the combination of 5-FU with nitrosoureas or a combination of 5-FU, adriamycin and mitomycin C (Kovach et al. 1974; MacDonald et al. 1979). In 1976 we decided to conduct a randomized trial with 5-FU/BCNU combination chemotherapy following curative gastric resection (Schlag et al. 1982). The recent results of our study are presented briefly below.

In this trial patients were stratified by tumor stage and randomly assigned to a control or a chemotherapy group. Eight chemotherapy courses each lasting 5 days were administered at

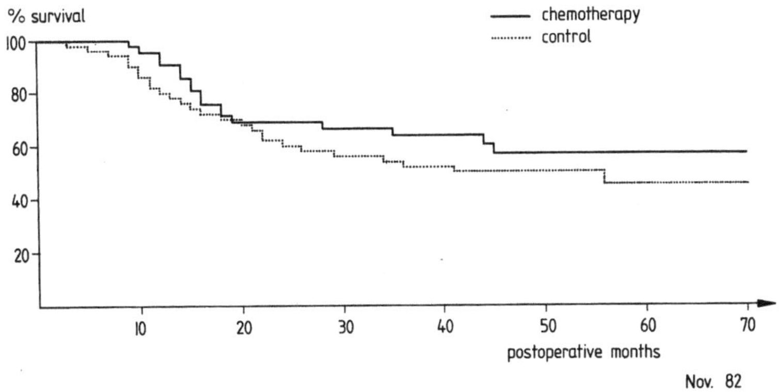

Fig. 1. Adjuvant 5-FU/BCNU trial in gastric cancer

6- to 9-week intervals. 5-FU was given IV at a dosage of 10 mg/kg daily and BCNU was given at a dosage of 40 mg/m^2 daily. There are 103 patients in this study: 54 in the control group and 49 randomized to the chemotherapy arm. After an observation period of 5 years, comparison of the survival time shows no statistical difference between the groups of treated and untreated patients (Fig. 1). There is no statistically proven benefit for the treatment group. The probability of survival was 50% in the control arm and 57% in the group of patients randomized to chemotherapy. The distribution of the total of 45 relapses is revealing. Adjuvant therapy had no effect on the frequency of local relapse or on the occurrence of distant metastases. Further analysis of the data shows the expected better prognosis for patients in tumor stage II in comparison with stage III. When the control and treatment arms in both subsets of patients are compared no prognostic benefit can be observed. Therefore, the analysis of our trial does not demonstrate a statistically proven benefit of adjuvant 5-FU and BCNU treatment in the dosage and schedule used following curative resection of gastric cancer. A final assessment of this surgical adjuvant approach must also await the results of other trials currently in progress to investigate a similar concept (Table 5). Recently the Gastrointestinal Tumor Study Group has reported a positive result with adjuvant 5-FU and methyl-CCNU chemotherapy (Gastrointestinal Tumor Study Group 1982). Nevertheless, the difference in survival for the whole group reached only borderline significance. The number of patients that had to be removed from the study was relatively high, with 23 out of 165. As these patients were not included in the

Table 5. Controlled trials of perioperative chemotherapy following curative resection for gastric cancer: Postoperative long-term single-agent chemotherapy

Group	Number of patients	Drug	Survival benefit for treated patients
Hattori et al. (1976)	278	Mitomycin C	No improvement
Fujimoto et al. (1977)	107	5-FU	Significant improvement
Koyama (1978)	318	Mitomycin C	No improvement
	159	5-FU	No improvement
	101	TSPA	No improvement
	141	CX-CM	No improvement

final evaluation the more favorable outcome of the study may be partly explained. Accordingly, other trials with combination chemotherapy performed by the Eastern Cooperative Oncology Group, the VASOG, and others have not yet proved differences in prognosis between control and adjuvant therapy groups in accordance with our results (Blake et al. 1981; Engström et al. 1981; Higgins 1979). Furthermore, the side-effects that occurred in some of the chemotherapy patients must also be mentioned. In our study half of this patient group complained of relatively severe gastrointestinal distress, such as nausea, vomiting, and diarrhea, in connection with the therapy performed. Adjuvant 5-FU/BCNU treatment had to be modified in our study in 17 of 42 patients and discontinued in 4 of them because of persisting hematological side-effects.

In our study, particular attention has been paid to these haematological side-effects. It has been shown that the circulating granulopoietic stem cells may be a particularly sensitive indicator for a prolonged defect in granulopoiesis (Lohrmann et al. 1982).

In conclusion, the question arises as to whether the failure of perioperative or adjuvant chemotherapy in gastric carcinoma is due ultimately to the lack of effectiveness of the cytostatic drugs available at the present time or to inappropriate concepts in treatment planning. Perioperative and adjuvant chemotherapy in gastric cancer is far from being generally recommended. At the moment the legitimate desire to improve a patient's survival chance should not lead to the advocation and use of a treatment modality that seems promising in theory but is in reality ineffective and gives rise to additional adverse effects in the patients.

References

Blake IRS, Hardcastle JD, Wilson RG (1981) Gastric cancer: a controlled trial of adjuvant chemotherapy following gastrectomy. Clin Oncol 7: 13–21

Burchenal JH (1976) Adjuvant therapy – theory, practis and potential. Cancer 37: 46–57

Dent DM, Werner ID, Novis B, Cheverton P, Brice P (1979) Prospective randomized trial of combined oncological therapy for gastric carcinoma. Cancer 44: 385–391

Dixon WJ, Longmire WP Jr, Holden WD (1971) Use of triethylenthiophosphoramide as an adjuvant to the surgical treatment of gastric and colorectal carcinoma: ten-year follow-up. Ann Surg 173: 26–34

Dwight RW, Humphrey EW, Higgins GA (1973) FUDR as an adjuvant to surgery in cancer of the large bowel. J Surg Oncol 5: 243–249

Engström PF, Lavin P, Douglass HO Jr (1981) Adjuvant therapy of gastric carcinoma using 5-fluorouracil (5FU) plus semustine (meCCNU): a preliminary report. In: Gerard A (ed) Progress and perspectives in the treatment of gastrointestinal tumors. Pergamon, Oxford, pp 31–35

Fujimoto S (1976) A study of survival in patients with stomach cancer treated by a combination of preoperative intra-arterial infusion therapy and surgery. Cancer 37: 1648–1653

Fujimoto S (1977) Protracted oral chemotherapy with fluorinated pyrimidines as an adjuvant to surgical treatment for stomach cancer. Ann Surg 185: 462–466

Gastrointestinal Tumor Study Group (1982) Controlled trial of adjuvant chemotherapy following curative resection for gastric cancer. Cancer 49: 1116–1122

Goffin IC (1978) Adjuvant therapy of gastric cancer. The 40742 clinical trial of the EORTC Gastro-Intestinal Tract Cooperative Group. In: Gerard A (ed) Gastro-intestinal tumors: a clinical and experimental approach. Pergamon, Oxford, pp 27–29

Hattori T, Mori A, Hirata K, Ito I (1972) Five-year survival rate of gastric cancer patients treated by gastrectomy, large dose of mitomycin C and/or allogeneic bone marrow transplantation. Gan 63: 517–522

Herfarth Ch, Schlag P (1979) Gastric cancer. Springer, Berlin Heidelberg New York

Higgins GA (1979) Chemotherapy in advanced gastric cancer. In: Herfarth Ch, Schlag P (eds) Gastric cancer. Springer, Berlin Heidelberg New York, pp 361–366

Higgins GA, Flynn T, Gillespie J (1964) Effect of splenectomy on tolerance to thio-TEPA. Arch Surg 88: 627–632

Imanaga H, Nakazato H (1977) Results of surgery for gastric cancer and effect of adjuvant mitomycin C on cancer recurrence. Worls J Surg 1: 213–221

Jinnai D, Higashi H (1976) Extended radical operation with preoperative chemotherapy for gastric cancer. Gan 18: 111–119

Kovach JS, Moertel CG, Schutt AJ, Hahn RG, Reitemeir RJ (1974) A controlled study of combined 1, 3- bis-(2-chlorethyl)-1-nitrosurea and 5-fluorouracil therapy for advanced gastric and pancreatic cancer. Cancer 33: 563–567

Koyama Y (1978) The current status of chemotherapy for gastric cancer in Japan with special emphasis on mitomycin C. Recent Results Cancer Res 63: 135–147

Lohrmann HP, Lepp KA, Schreml W (1982) 5-fluorouracil, 1, 3-Bis (2-chloroethyl)-1-nitrosourea, and 1-(2-chloroethyl)-3-(4-methylcyclohexyl)-1-nitrosourea: effect on the human granulopoietic system. JNCI 68: 541–547

Longmire WP, Kuzma JW, Dixon WJ (1968) The use of triethylenethiophosphoramide as an adjuvant to the surgical treatment of gastric carcinoma. Ann Surg 167: 293–312

MacDonald JS, Wooley PV, Smythe T, Ueno W, Hoth D, Schein PS (1979) 5-fluorouracil, adriamycin and mitomycin C (FAM) combination chemotherapy in the treatment of advanced gastric cancer. Cancer 44: 42–47

Schlag P, Merkle P, Herfarth Ch (1979) Neue Aspekte in der Konzeption adjuvanter und nachsorgender Therapie des Magencarcinoms? Chirurg 50: 432–435

Schlag P, Schreml W, Gaus W, Herfarth CH, Linder MM, Queisser W, Trede M (1982) Adjuvant 5-fluorouracil and BCNU chemotherapy in gastric cancer: 3-year results. Recent Results Cancer Res 80: 277–283

Serlin O, Wolkoff JS, Amadeo JM, Keehn RJ (1969) Use of 5-fluorodesoxyuridine (FUDR) as an adjuvant to the surgical management of carcinoma of the stomach. Cancer 24: 224–228

The Risks of Perioperative Chemotherapy in Large-Bowel Cancer Surgery

U. Metzger

Chirurgische Onkologie, Departement Chirurgie, Universitätklinik,
8091 Zürich, Switzerland

Introduction

The approach of administering perioperative chemotherapy as an adjuvant to curative surgery in large-bowel cancer is really not a modern one, as it might seem to be today. Based on the observation of free malignant cells circulating in the blood during operation (Fisher and Turnbull 1955; Moore et al. 1957), several attemps have been made to treat these cancer cells prophylactically at the time of operation. In the mid-1950s, Warren Cole's group in Chicago initiated the idea of perioperative chemotherapy (Morales et al. 1957), supposing that cancer cells might be more vulnerable to the action of anticancer agents if given on the day of the operation, before these "loose" cells develop a blood supply. They stated: "Improvement in the 5-year survival rate of the surgical treatment of cancer during the past 10 or 15 years has been made primarily by increasing the extent of the operation. However, there is no hope that further improvement can be expected from this phase of the operation, because we are now approaching anatomical limits in respect to the amount of tissue that can be removed." This may still be true today. Following experimental research in rats, in March 1956 Cole's group started the clinical use of nitrogen mustard given to patients at the time of operation. A dose of 0.1 mg/kg body weight was given both through the portal venous system and into the peritoneal cavity during operation, and then IV on postoperative days 1 and 2. In a subsequent prospective randomized study (Mrazek et al. 1959) in patients with breast and large-bowel cancer, administration of nitrogen mustard resulted in significant bone marrow depression and resultant leukopenia varying in intensity in the majority of patients, particularly in elderly and obese patients. Minor and major complications occurred in 46% of the treated patients and 43.3% of the controls. The postoperative hospital stay was significantly longer in the treated group, especially in elderly patients, indicating that it might be more difficult to control a serious infection or hemorrhage during drug-induced pancytopenia.

Mitomen chemotherapy was given in 87 patients with carcinoma of the abdominal organs (Blixenkrone 1959), the drug being administered directly into the peritoneal cavity and IV during the immediate postoperative period up to a total dose of 600–700 mg. This treatment resulted in an unacceptably high hematological and neurological toxicity and was not recommended for further use.

The first cooperative clinical trial combining chemotherapy as an adjuvant to the surgical treatment of bowel cancer was reported by Holden et al. 1967, who administered thio-TEPA in the immediate postoperative period, 0.2 mg/kg given both IP and IV at

Recent Results in Cancer Research. Vol. 98

surgery and again the same dose IV on each of days 1 and 2 after surgery. There was some suggestion of beneficial effect in part I of the study, in which a total dose of 0.8 mg/kg was given; this was subsequently reduced to 0.6 mg/kg due to a rather high incidence of complications. A general recommendation of adjuvant therapy with alkylating agents was never made on the basis of this particular study. A similar study comparing perioperative thio-TEPA with untreated controls was conducted by the early Veterans Administration Surgical Adjuvant Group and revealed no difference in morbidity, mortality, or survival (Dwight et al. 1969).

The reported 20% response to fluorouracil chemotherapy (Rousselot et al. 1967) led to the development of a technique for giving intraluminal fluorouracil into the isolated bowel lumen at the time of surgical resection. A 10% complication rate has been reported, as against 19% in historical controls. The subsequent prospective randomized study (Grossi et al. 1977) revealed a postoperative complication rate of 23% in the control group and 27% in the fluorouracil-treated group. The postoperative hospital mortality figures were 6 of 242 in the control group (2.5%) and 7 of 264 in the fluorouracil-treated group (2.8%). Life-table analysis of survival in this study did not demonstrate a statistically significant difference.

A very similar study using intraluminal and IV chemotherapy at the time of operation has been conducted by Lawrence et al. (1975). In this prospective randomized trial patients were assigned to control or to 5-FU (30 mg per kg body weight) diluted in 50 ml physiologic saline and injected into the bowel lumen after colonic dissection with blood supply to the isolated colon ligated 30 minutes after intraluminal instillation. These patients also received IV 5-FU (10 mg per kg body weight) on the first and second postoperative days. Additional oral 5-FU was later given for a total of 1 year. Postoperative complications and operative mortality have been quite similar in this trial and – unfortunately, the disease-free and overall survival curves also do not differ significantly.

In a Veterans Administration Study, 5-FUDR was used in the perioperative period (Dwight et al. 1973): patients randomized to the treatment group were given a dose of 20 mg/kg of body weight with a maximum dose of 1.7 g IV as a single dose on each of the first, second, and third postoperative days. The second course was to be five doses of 30 mg/kg body weight, to be started preferably between the 35th and 45th postoperative days. The chemotherapy did not influence the total number of postoperative complications, but there were greater numbers of pulmonary complications in the treated patients (16.8% against 9.9% for the controls). No explanation has been found for this. The 30-day postoperative mortality for the two groups did not differ significantly but it was slightly lower for the control patients. The 5-year survival following curative resection was 47.1% for treated patients and 50.7% for the controls.

Systemic therapy with 5-FU alone or in combination has been used in many other studies (Higgins et al. 1967, 1971; Grage et al. 1977; Panettiere 1980; Killen et al. 1981; Mittelman et al. 1981). In these trials, the first chemotherapy was usually started 2 or more weeks postoperatively and repeated in 4–8 weeks. A 30% complication rate was reported in the Higgins study, but again there was no difference between the treatment and the control groups. Due to the late onset of adjuvant chemotherapy in these trials they cannot be considered as true perioperative chemotherapy studies.

In the late 1970s the lack of efficient systemic treatment of large-bowel cancer again stimulated the localized approach to the presumable site of recurrence. In more recent studies conducted in the United Kingdom and in Switzerland, the portal venous route was used for continued early postoperative liver perfusion. In a prospective randomized study, Taylor et al. (1979) investigated the influence of 1 g 5-FU given by continuous administration through an umbilical vein catheter during the first postoperative week. A slight decrease in white cell count on days 6 and 8 was observed, whereas postoperative morbidity and mortality were not influenced by this regional chemotherapy. In a similar study conducted by the Swiss Group for Clinical Cancer Research, a daily perfusion of 5-FU 500 mg per m^2 for the first 7 postoperative days with a mitomycin-C bolus (10 mg per m^2) on day 1 is used. Again a slight decrease in leukocyte count was observed in three patients with nadirs of 1,600, 2,200, and 2,300 per m^3 between days 10 and 14. Morbidity and duration of hospital stay were similar in the treated and control groups, with two deaths in the whole series of 110 patients, being one death in each group.

Conclusions

1. Due to the lack of efficient systemic treatment, current adjuvant efforts in large-bowel cancer are directed at the presumed site of recurrence.
2. These localized approaches are probably less burdened with systemic side-effects and therefore suitable for perioperative treatment. Results of ongoing cooperative trials using radiotherapy, liver perfusion, or the "belly bath" technique are awaited with interest.
3. If severe side-effects are expected, perioperative chemotherapy should be delayed for a period of at least 8–10 days because it would obviously be more difficult to control a serious infection or hemorrhage in large-bowel surgery during drug-induced pancytopenia.
4. Finally, all adjuvant treatment of large-bowel cancer is still experimental and should be restricted to prospective controlled studies.

References

Blixenkrone N (1959) Mitomen cheotherapy given in relation to operation for cancer of the abdominal organs. Acta Chir Scand 117: 189–196

Dwight RW, Higgins GA, Keehn RJ (1969) Factors influencing survival after resection in cancer of the colon and rectum. Am J Surg 117: 512–522

Dwight RW, Humphrey EW, Higgins GA, Keehn RJ (1973) FUDR as an adjuvant to surgery in cancer of the large bowel. J Surg Oncol 5: 243–249

Fisher ER, Turnbull RB (1955) The cytological demonstration and significance of tumor cells in the mesenteric venous blood in patients with colorectal cancer. Surg Gynecol Obstet 100: 102–108

Grage TB, Metter GE, Cornell GN, Strawitz JG, Hill GJ, Frelick RW, Moss SE (1977) Adjuvant chemotherapy with 5-Fluorouracil after surgical resection of colorectal carcinoma (COG Protocol 7041). A preliminary report. Am J Surg 133: 59–66

Grossi CE, Wolff WI, Nealon TF, Pasternack B, Ginzburg L, Rousselot LM (1977) Intraluminal fluorouracil chemotherapy adjunct to surgical procedures for resectable carcinoma of the colon and rectum. Surg Gynecol Obstet 145: 549–554

Higgins GA, Dwight RW, Swith JV, Keehn RJ (1971) Fluorouracil as an adjuvant to surgery in carcinoma of the colon. Arch Surg 102: 339–343

Higgins GA, Humphrey E, Juler GL, LeVeen HH, McCaughan J, Keehn RJ (1976) Adjuvant chemotherapy in the surgical treatment of large bowel cancer. Cancer 38: 1461–1467

Holden WD, Dixon WJ, Kuzma JW (1967) The use of triethylenethiophosphoramide as an adjuvant to the surgical treatment of colorectal carcinoma. Ann Surg 165: 481–491

Killen JY, Holyoke ED, Moertel CG, Horton J, Schein PS, Ellenberg SS (1981) Adjuvant therapy of adenocarcinoma of the colon following clinically curative resection: an interim report from the GITSG In: Jones SE, Salmon SE (eds) Adjuvant therapy of cancer III. Grune and Stratton, New York, pp 527–538

Lawrence W, Terz JJ, Horsley S, Donaldson M, Lovett WL, Brown PW, Ruffner BW, Regelson W (1975) Chemotherapy as an adjuvant to surgery for colorectal cancer. Ann Surg 181:616–623

Mittelman A, Moertal CG, Horton J, Levin B, Schein PS, Novak JW (1981) Adjuvant chemotherapy and radiotherapy following rectal surgery: an interim report from the GITSG. In: Jones SE, Salmon SE (eds) Adjuvant therapy of Cancer III. Grune and Stratton, New York, pp 547–557

Moore GE, Sandberg A, Schubarg JR (1957) Clinical and experimental observations of the occurrence and fate of tumor cells in the blood stream. Ann Surg 146:580–587

Morales F, Bell M, McDonald G, Cole WH (1957) The prophylactic treatment of cancer at the time of operation. Ann Surg 146:588–595

Mrazek R, Economou S, McDonald G, Slaughter P, Cole WH (1959) Prophylactic and adjuvant use of nitrogen mustard in the surgical treatment of cancer. Ann Surg 150:745–755

Panettiere FJ (1980) Adjuvant chemotherapy with or without immunotherapy in colorectal cancer. Clin Res 28(5):837A

Rousselot LM, Cole DR, Grossi CE, Conte AJ, Gonzales EM (1967) Intraluminal chemotherapy (HN2 or 5-FU) adjuvant to operation for cancer of the colon and rectum. II. Follow-up report of 97 cases. Cancer 20:829–833

Taylor I, Rowling JT, West C (1979) Adjuvant cytotoxic liver perfusion for colorectal cancer. Br J Surg 66:833–837

The Need for Pilot Studies and Surgery-Only Controls in Adjuvant Therapy Trials for Large-Bowel Cancer

W. Weber-Stadelmann*

Heuberg 16, 4051 Basel, Switzerland

Introduction

The object of clinical treatment research is to discover new methods of therapy which will improve therapeutic results, the survival of cancer patients, and/or the quality of survival. The methodology used is that of the clinical trial. A successful clinical trial which shows that a new treatment approach is superior to standard techniques can have enormous implications for medical practice. Currently systemic adjuvant therapy with cytostatic drugs is being evaluated in a wide range of human malignancies. If these adjuvant therapies are proven to be beneficial then every patient with certain stages of breast cancer, bowel cancer, lung cancer, etc. will routinely be asked to undergo additional therapy after surgery. Patients and the public view clinical trials as important, ethical, and as a means of attaining superior clinical care (Cassileth et al. 1982).

Material, Methods, and Results

The Disease-Oriented Committee for Gastrointestinal Cancer of the Swiss Group for Clinical Cancer Research (SAKK) decided at its first meeting in October 1979, after an indepth analysis of the historical data base, to embark on a clinical study of adjuvant liver perfusion with 5-fluorouracil (FU) and mitomycin C (MM) starting immediately after complete resection of colorectal adenocarcinoma. No similar study had ever been done in this country before. We were hesitant to start a large multicenter trial without some preliminary data generated by the prospective study participants. It was therefore decided to do a *pilot trial* (Fig. 1). Within 6 months, 20 evaluable patients were treated in five of the seven Swiss centers. The major postoperative morbidity found took the form of infections and anastomotic dehiscence (Table 1). From this first experience the following impression emerged:

1. Postoperative 7-day FU and MMC liver perfusion through the portal vein can be performed in the majority of the prospective study centers.
2. The expected major postoperative morbidity will probably consist in infections and anastomotic dehiscence.

* For the Swiss Group for Clinical Cancer Research

Recent Results in Cancer Research. Vol. 98

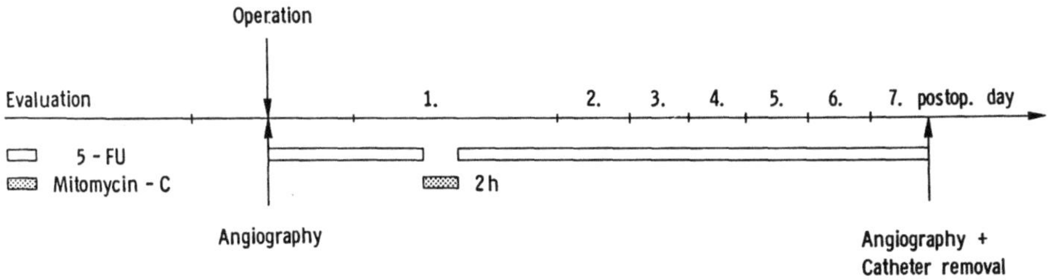

Fig. 1. Schedule of the SAKK 40/81 pilot study

The pilot study initiated intensive discussions and consultations between the investigators on technical problems. This led to the acceptance of standard criteria for pre-, peri-, and postoperative measures (e.g., bowel preparation, antibiotics, type of catheter).
A *phase III study* was then initiated with an increased degree of confidence in its practicability in June 1981. It is a prospective, randomized, and controlled trial (Fig. 2). 79 patients entered the study in the first year. Major toxicities were infections and anastomotic dehiscence in both the chemotherapy and the surgery-only groups (Table 2). The incidence and spectrum of toxicity are comparable to those in the pilot study (Table 3). So far there is no difference in morbidity between the adjuvant chemotherapy arm and the surgery-only arm.

Discussion and Conclusions

On the basis of experience with a trial of adjuvant liver FU and MMC perfusion in colorectal adenocarcinoma the need for a *pilot study* can be summarized as follows:

1. Exploration of practicability and potential morbidity of a new treatment modality in a relatively small number of patients.
2. Test of the potential patient accrual and interest of the prospective investigators.
3. Standardization of procedures and exercise in cooperative work.

Such a pilot study can enhance the chance of success of a subsequent large clinical trial.

Table 1. SAKK 40/81 pilot study of adjuvant liver perfusion (5-FU + MMC) in 20 patients (13 male, 7 female; median age: 62 years; range: 41–74)

Postoperative morbidity	Patients	
	n	%
Infection (wound, drainage channel)	3	15
Anastomotic dehiscence	1	5
Stomatitis (1+)	1	5
Total	5	25

Leukopenia: 1 patient (3,600/mm^3)

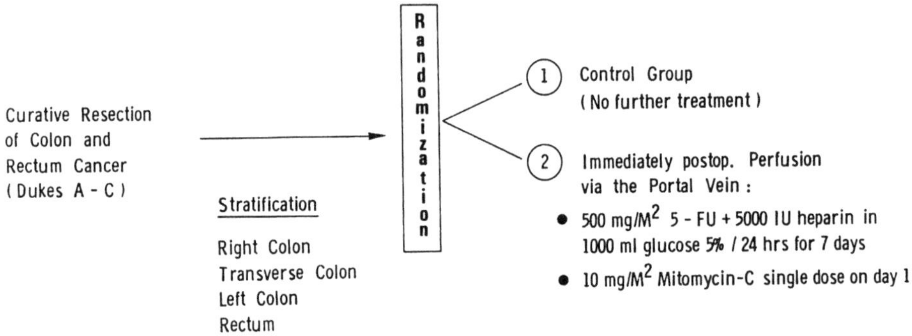

Fig. 2. Schedule for the SAKK 40/81 phase III study

Table 2. SAKK 40/81 prospective, randomized phase III study on adjuvant liver perfusion (5-FU + MMC), preliminary data on the first 79 patients

Postoperative morbidity	Surgery + perfusion $n = 41$ (23 m, 18 f) Median age: 62 years (Range: 40–74)		Surgery only $n = 38$ (20 m, 18 f) Median age: 62 years (Range: 43–77)	
	n	%	*n*	%
Infection (wound, drainage channel)	4	10	6	16
Anastomotic dehiscence	3	7	2	5
Persistent perineal sinus	2	5	0	
Small-bowel obstruction	1		1	
Hemorrhage	0		1	
Thrombosis/embolism	1		1	
Total	11	27	11	29
Leukopenia:	2 patients (1,600, 2,200/mm^3)			

Table 3. SAKK 40/81: Comparison of postoperative morbidity between pilot and phase III study

Postoperative morbidity	Pilot study		Randomized study			
	Surgery + perfusion		Surgery + perfusion		Sugery only	
	n	%	*n*	%	*n*	%
Infection	3	15	4	10	6	16
Anastomotic dehiscence	1	5	3	7	2	5
Stomatitis	1		0		0	
Persistent sinus	0		2		0	
Small-bowell obstruction	0		1		1	
Hemorrhage	0		0		1	
Thrombosis/embolism	0		1		1	
Total	5	25	11	27	11	29

Pilot studies are not suitable for testing efficacy of a new treatment, for reasons given by Spodick (1982). The *randomized controlled clinical trial* (RCT) has become the accepted standard means of demonstrating the true therapeutic effects and evaluating most forms of treatment. Its scientific and ethical bases are well established. In nonrandomized studies systematic nonrandom biases could well exist, and in many cases these biases are large enough to be medically misleading (Peto 1978). Carter (1980) has described the following characteristics of adjuvant trials:

- Microscopic foci of metastatic disease are treated, which are assumed from theoretical assumptions to be present, but which cannot be seen, measured, or evaluated except indirectly in terms of ultimate relapse and survival.
- Long-term analysis is a sine qua non.
- Objective regression or response cannot be used to aid the assessment.
- The first end-point is the relapse rate, from which an actuarial projection of a relapse-free survival curve can be constructed.
- The first available cost-benefit analysis is between relapse rate and acute toxicity. What is not known at this time is the minimum duration of follow-up needed to ensure that an actuarial projection of a relapse-free survival based on relapse rates at early fixed time points will predict the ultimate outcome.

The evaluation of morbidity in the first 79 patients of the SAKK 40/81 study illustrates how important the addition of a surgery-only arm is. Fear that a new treatment will add additional risk is a major behavioral pitfall of physicians (Spodick 1982). This fear should be a major reason *for* randomized clinical trials (RCTs): these give a patient a "50–50 chance" of not being exposed to a trial treatment (Spodick 1982). It is reassuring for the continuation of the study that spectrum and incidence of postoperative morbidity has not been changed so far by the addition of postoperative FU and MMC liver perfusion.

References

Carter SK (1980) Clinical considerations in the design of clinical trials. Cancer Treat Rep 64:367–371

Cassileth BR, Lusk EJ, Miller DS, Hurwitz S (1982) Attitudes toward clinical trials among patients and the public. JAMA 248:968–970

Peto R (1978) Clinical trial methodology. Biomedicine [Special Issue] 28:24–36

Spodick DH (1982) Randomized controlled clinical trials. The behavioral case. JAMA 247:2258–2260

Clinical Experience with Preoperative Chemotherapy for Osteosarcoma

H. P. Honegger, M. Cserhati, A. R. von Hochstetter, V. Hofmann, and P. Groscurth

FMH Innere Medizin (speziell Hämatologie), Stadtspital Triemli, 8063 Zürich, Switzerland

Introduction

Since 1978, patients with osteosarcomas have been treated with preoperative chemotherapy (Cserhati et al. 1981). As an additional and important part of our bone sarcoma studies in Zurich, we transplant specimens obtained at the initial biopsy and at the resection after chemotherapy into nude mice for additional evaluation (Groscurth et al. 1982). Several experimental essays for chemosensitivity testing are then performed, as has been outlined elsewhere (Hofmann et al. 1983). An essential and important part is the evaluation by conventional histological analysis and the measurement of necrotic changes in the resected tumors. Our technique for assessment of necrosis has been described elsewhere (Von Hochstetter et al. 1981).

Materials and Methods

From 1978 to 1982 a consecutive series of 15 patients with histologically confirmed osteosarcomas was admitted to our study, regardless of age or location of the primary tumor. There were 10 male and 5 female patients. One patient already had lung metastasis at presentation with the primary tumor. In 2 patients new lung metastases were diagnosed after resection of their primary tumors without additional chemotherapy. They were then treated with preoperative chemotherapy before undergoing thoracotomy for resection of their metastases. The other patients presented with primary tumors only.

Nine patients were treated according to the T7 protocol, and six according to the T10 protocol. The T7 chemotherapy protocol involves high-dose methotrexate (HDMTX) with vincristine and citrovorum factor (Leucovorin) rescue and cyclophosphamide, bleomycin plus dactinomycin and adriamycin (Rosen et al. 1979). The T10 chemotherapy protocol relies entirely on HDMTX plus vincristine and citrovorum factor (Leucovorin) rescue in the preoperative phase (Rosen et al. 1982a). HDMTX was administered following a strict protocol with hydration, alkalization of the urine, and citrovorum factor rescue. Serum levels of MTX were measured at 24 and 48 hours.

For the final analysis we divided our material into two groups. Group A refers to patients who showed little or no necrosis after preoperative chemotherapy (less than 50% by definition). Group B consists of patients who had markedly over 50% necrosis in their resected tumors.

Recent Results in Cancer Research. Vol. 98

After resection of the tumor, chemotherapy is completed and patients are then followed at our outpatient clinics. Relapse-free survival and overall survival are calculated from the date of histological analysis after preoperative chemotherapy and are shown according to the method of Kaplan and Meyer (1958). For comparison of groups A and B the log rank test was used (Peto et al. 1977).

Results

Tolerance of Preoperative Chemotherapy

Significant changes in terms of hemoglobin level, white blood cell count, and platelet counts were not observed between initiation of preoperative chemotherapy and surgical intervention.

An overview of the side-effects seen during preoperative chemotherapy is given in Table 1. Mucositis occurred mostly in patients treated according to the T7-chemotherapy protocol. Patients treated with the T10 protocol, i.e., with successive administrations of HDMTX, sometimes experienced pleuritic pain. Signs of neurotoxicity were also seen in T10 patients; these included headaches and paresthesias, occasionally with pleocytosis in the CNS fluid. One case of transient, fully reversible paresis of the 9th cranial nerve was observed. In patients treated according to the T7 chemotherapy protocol, especially, these side-effects caused further chemotherapy to be delayed. In both groups A and B, however, these delays were evenly distributed. The T10 protocol was applied according to the outline of Rosen (1982a) without delay.

Preoperative chemotherapy did not have any impact on the surgical procedures. The postoperative course was felt to be normal with respect to wound healing and mobilization of the patient, and no infections were seen. Surgical procedures included amputations or resections of primary tumors with preservation of the limb.

Survival

Using the extent of necrosis, we divided our material in two groups and analyzed them retrospectively. Group A consisted of seven patients who had less than 50% necrosis after

Table 1. Side-effects

Effect	Group			
	A		B	
	T−7	T−10	T−7	T−10
Mucositis	6	0	2	1
Fever	6	1	0	1
Pain	1	0	0	3
Neurological	0	1	1	4
Totals	15		12	

preoperative chemotherapy. Group B refers to eight patients who had much more than 50% necrosis in their resected tumors. Relapse-free survival is significantly better for group B (Fig. 1) than for group A. In terms of relapse-free survival, patients in group A roughly follow the course of a historical group of patients treated in our institutions with amputation only without additional chemotherapy. Figure 2 shows the overall survival of the two groups, and again, patients in group B survive longer than those in group A. All patients treated since 1978 with additional chemotherapy seem to fare better than those in the historical group without chemotherapy, at least during the first 12–18 months.

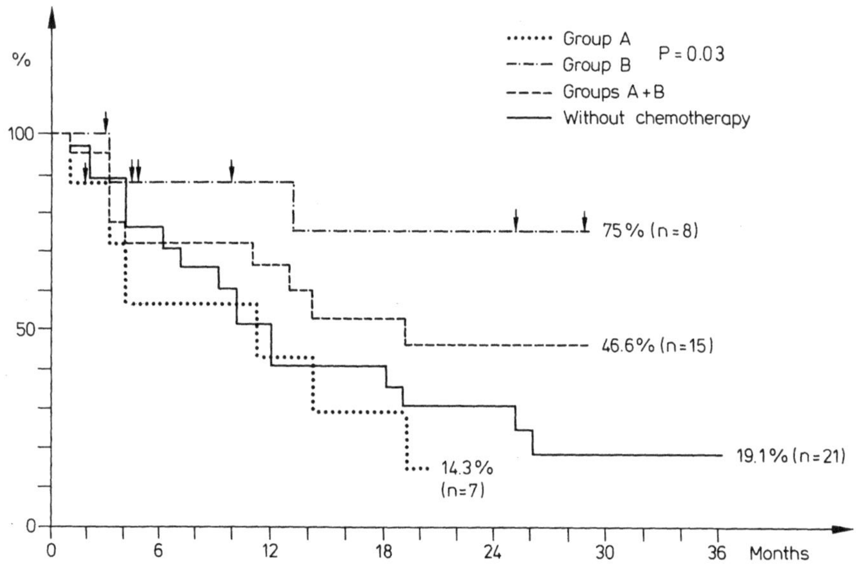

Fig. 1. Kaplan-Meier estimated relapse curves

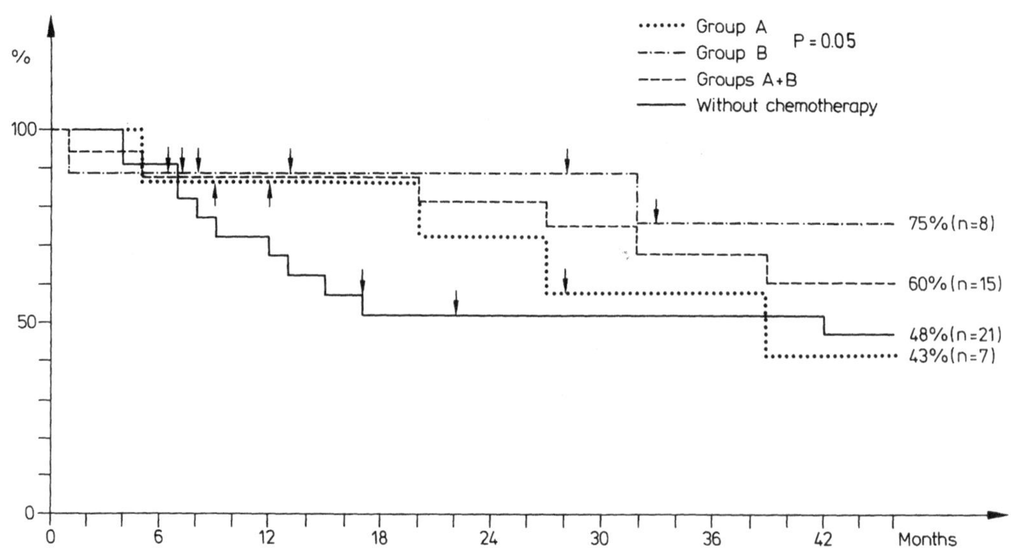

Fig. 2. Kaplan-Meier estimated survival curves

Discussion

In our small study of 15 patients with osteosarcomas, preoperative chemotherapy was acceptably well tolerated and did not impair surgical procedures. Postoperative wound healing was normal despite preoperative chemotherapy, and no infections were observed among our patients. HDMTX was administered with no major problems, and renal function was not disturbed in any case. Due to the side-effects mentioned above, we were not able to proceed with the T7 chemotherapy protocol as outlined by Rosen (1979). These side-effects sometimes caused delays with further chemotherapy. The T10 chemotherapy protocol, on the other hand, was given according to the outline of Rosen (1982a) with no delays.

The achievement and the extent of necrosis after preoperative chemotherapy are considered important indicators for the biological course of the disease by several groups (Huvos 1977; Rosen 1979). Our small retrospective analysis confirms that patients with extensive necrosis after preoperative chemotherapy (= group B) do indeed have a lower relapse rate and a longer overall survival than those with little necrosis (= group A). The extent of necrosis after preoperative chemotherapy may thus be used as a parameter for the effectiveness of preoperative chemotherapy; in cases with no evidence of necrosis other chemotherapeutic agents than those used in the T7 or T10 chemotherapy protocols should probably be recommended (Rosen 1982). However, further investigations concerning the impact of necrosis are urgently needed, since the incidence of spontaneous necrosis in untreated osteosarcomas is still largely unknown.

Our small study does not allow a comparison of the effectiveness of different treatment regimens, nor does it yield further information with respect to the real impact of HDMTX in the management of osteosarcomas. An ongoing study with the patients randomized between surgery only and preoperative chemotherapy according to the T10 chemotherapy protocol will provide us with important information in this respect (Lange 1982).

Summary

Since 1978 preoperative chemotherapy has been administered to 15 consecutive patients with osteosarcomas in Zurich. Preoperative chemotherapy was acceptably well tolerated and did not impair surgical procedures. Our retrospective analysis confirmed that the extent of necrosis after preoperative chemotherapy is of biological importance for the further course of the disease. Patients with extensive necrosis had better relapse-free survival and longer overall survival than those with little necrosis.

References

Cserhati M, Honegger HP, von Hochstetter A, Groscurth P, Hofmann V (1983) Zurich bone sarcome study I. Concepts of the clinical, morphological and functional study. In: Verhandlungen der deutschen Krebsgesellschaft, Vol 4, Fischer, Stuttgart, p 782

Groscurth P, Hofmann V, Cserhati M, von Hochstetter A, Honegger HP (1982) Xenogeneic transplantation and in vitro cultivation of human osteosarcomas after preoperative chemotherapy. Proceedings of the 13th international cancer congress, Sept 13. Abstract 2159, p 379

Honegger HP, von Hochstetter A, Groscurth P, Hofmann V, Cserhati M (1984) The effect of chemotherapy on human bone sarcomas: a clinical and experimental study. In: Hofmann V,

Berens ME, Martz G (eds) Predictive drug testing on human tumor cells. Springer, Berlin Heidelberg New York Tokyo, p 65. In: Recent results in cancer research, Vol 94

Huvos AG, Rosen G, Marcove RL (1977) Primary osteogenic sarcoma. Pathologic aspects in 20 patients after treatment with chemotherapy, en bloc resection and prosthetic bone replacement. Arch Pathol Lab Med 101:14

Kaplan EZ, Meier P (1958) Non parametric estimation für incomplete observations. J Am Statist Assoc 53:457

Lange B, Levine AS (1982) Is it ethical not to conduct a prospectively controlled trial of adjuvant chemotherapy in osteosarcoma? Cancer Treat Rep 66:1699

Peto R, Pike M, Armitage P (1977) Design and analysis of randomized clinical trials requiring prolonged observation of each patient. II. Analysis and examples. Br J Cancer 35:1

Rosen G, Marcove R, Caparros B, Nirenberg A, Kosloff C, Huvos A (1979) Primary osteogenic sarcoma. The rationale for preoperative chemotherapy and delayed surgery. Cancer 43:2163

Rosen G, Caparros B, Huvos A, Kosloff C, Nirenberg A, Cacavio A, Marcove R, Lane J, Mehta B, Urban Ch (1982) Preoperative chemotherapy for osteogenic sarcoma. Cancer 19:1221

Rosen G, Caparros B, Nirenberg A. Cisplatinum-adriamycin combination chemotherapy in evaluable osteogenic sarcoma. Proc Am Soc Clin Oncol 1:173 (abstract C-672)

Effect of Intensive Adjuvant Chemotherapy on Wound Healing in 69 Patients with Osteogenic Sarcomas of the Lower Extremities

O. Bertermann, R. C. Marcove, and G. Rosen

Klinikum rechts der Isar, Chirurgie, Station I/17,
Ismaninger Strasse 22, 8000 München 22, Germany

Introduction

Survival time and quality of life can be increased in patients with osteogenic sarcomas by means of preoperative chemotherapy and en-bloc resection (Rosen and Nirenberg 1982). Rosen et al. (1982) reported that 53 of 57 patients (93%) with osteogenic sarcoma had no evidence of recurrence or metastatic disease at 6–35 months (median 20 months) from the start of treatment.

With the advent of aggressive adjuvant chemotherapy it has become important to characterize the effect of these powerful toxic agents on wound healing. These effects have been subjected to clinical observation and laboratory investigations (Graaves and Raaf 1980). Clinical impressions suggest that chemotherapeutic agents may interfere with wound healing. Normal defense mechanisms may be diminished or absent, possibly leading to an increased postoperative morbidity and mortality in these patients (Guthrie and Long 1979; Shamberger et al. 1981). The majority of reported surgical trials in humans using adjuvant chemotherapy have resulted in little clinically significant impairment of wound healing (Graaves and Raaf 1980). Often in such trials subtherapeutic doses are used or the drugs are administered relatively late in the wound healing process.

It is the objective of our retrospective study to investigate the effect of intensive pre- and postoperative chemotherapy on wound healing in patients with osteogenic sarcomas of the lower extremities.

Materials and Methods

Patients

This study includes patients with primary osteogenic sarcomas of the lower extremities. All histological subtypes of malignant osteogenic sarcomas were included. Five patients with a massive tumor were rejected for en-bloc resection. This series is also unique in that the procedure was carried out by the same surgeon in each case.

Between June 1974 and October 1981, in all 69 patients meeting the criteria were included in this study. The median age of the patients was 17 years, with a range of 11–31 years. There were 29 male and 40 female patients. In 34 patients a total femur replacement was performed. In 15 patients total knee replacement was performed for upper tibia and one

Recent Results in Cancer Research. Vol. 98

fibula with skip area into tibia. A further 20 patients had a long-stem Guépar knee replacement for distal femur lesions.

Surgery

Of the patients with lesions of the femur, 54 underwent resection and endoprosthetic replacement of the tumor-bearing portion of the femur and knee joint following preoperative chemotherapy. In 15 patients total knee replacements were inserted for upper tibia and one fibula with skip area into tibia. During surgery, the entire femur and knee were carefully resected, care being taken to resect the margin of normal tissue around the specimen at all times. The sciatic and popliteal nerves along with the popliteal artery branches were resected from the tumor mass. The quadriceps mechanism was preserved only when cleared from tumor. The patella was either removed or cut coronally so that the knee joint was removed intact en bloc, the entire femur transsection being just above the tibial tubercle. When the total femur was resected, the abductors of the hip were marked so that they could be reapproximated to the upper femur prosthesis. The prosthesis was then inserted into the distal tibia shaft, the stem being fixed with methyl methacrylate and the distal portion of the tibia. Abductors or hamstring muscles were frequently transferred into the quadriceps mechanisms or made to form a layer between the skin and metal in case of superficial wound infection.

Diagnostic Studies

All patients underwent a pretreatment evaluation, which included anteroposterior and lateral chest roentgenograms, roentgenograms of the primary lesion taken in two planes, technitium-99 bone scan, and biochemical profile including serum alkaline phosphatase, 24-h urine calcium, creatinine clearance, and either conventional tomography or computerized transaxial tomography of the chest to rule out the presence of pulmonary metastasis. All patients had frequent follow-up serum alkaline phosphatase assays and frequent physical examinations, which included measurement of the size of the primary tumor, determination of tenderness to palpation, and questioning about objective relief of pain during preoperative chemotherapy. After 4 weeks of high-dose methotrexate treatment all diagnostic studies were repeated.

Chemotherapy

Preoperative chemotherapy was administered according to the T4, T5, T7, or T10 protocol (Rosen et al. 1976; Table 1), usually in an outpatient setting. A detailed description of the chemotherapy protocol has been published previously (Rosen and Nirenberg 1982; Rosen et al. 1976, 1982; Altemeier et al. 1970). All patients received pre- and postoperative antibiotics. Cephalosporin and aminoglucosides were given in the majority of cases.

Table 1. Drugs used in the T4, T7, and T10 protocols

Protocol	Year	Drugs[b]
T4	1974	HDMTX + CFR, C, ADT
T7	1976	HDMTX + CFR, BCD, ADR
T10[a]	1978	HDMTX + CRF, BCD, ADR, CIS

[a] Rosen et al. 1982
[b] *HDMTX*, high-dose methotrexate; *CFR*, citrovorum factor rescue; *C*, cyclophosphamide; *ADR*, adriamycin; *CIS*, *cis*-platinum; *B*, bleomycin

Definitions

A wound was defined as infected if pus discharged from it. A wound was categorized as possibly infected if it developed signs of inflammation or serous drainage. Wounds were classified as clean, clean-contaminated, contaminated, or dirty.

Clean. This category included extremity wounds in which no apparent inflammation was encountered and in which no break in aseptic technique occurred.

Clean-contaminated. This category included clean operation wounds in which there was a break in technique.

Contaminated. This category included operation wounds in which acute inflammation was encountered.

Dirty. This category included operation wounds in which obvious pus was encountered. In all our cases, the infection was confirmed by positive cultures or the pathology report of purulent tissue.
Only the infections that required a secondary operative procedure were included in the study. Transient inflammation that resolved quickly with conservative treatment was not included.

Results

In 55 of 69 patients (80%) wound healing was uneventful. In 14 of the 69 patients (20%) a postoperative wound infection requiring a secondary operative procedure developed (Table 2). In 10 of the patients (14%) débridement with or without skin grafting had to be performed. In 4 of the patients (6%) amputation was necessary (Table 3). One amputation had to be performed at 3 months, the others at 4, 8, and 20 months postoperatively. All the

Table 2. Incidence of infection requiring secondary surgery in 69 patients with osteogenic sarcoma of the lower extremities

No postoperative infection	55/69	(80%)
Postoperative infection	14/69	(20%)

Table 3. Operative procedures in patients with postoperative wound infections and osteogenic sarcoma of the lower extremities

Debridement ± skin graft	10/69	(14%)
Amputation	4/69	(6%)

Table 4. Interval between primary surgery and amputation

Case	Year	Months after primary surgery
1	1/1975	3
2	4/1975	8
3	4/1977	20
4	6/1977	4

Table 5. Types of wound infection

Type	No.	(Proportion)
Mixed bacterial infection	13/14	(93%)
Fungal infection	1/14	(7%)

amputations were early in the series, 2 being performed in 1975 and the other 2 in 1977 (Table 4). One amputation had to be done in a patient (EV) who had received 66 Gy prior to surgery. Of 14 patients with infection, 9 required a secondary operative procedure during their hospital stay (1 amputation and 8 débridements, with and without skin grafts).

With regard to the type of infection no specific bacterium could be identified. After 13 of 14 operations (93%) mixed bacterial infections were found. One patient (EV) developed a fungal infection (Table 5). After secondary surgery wound healing was uneventful in most of our patients. No patient died as a consequence of wound infection. Infections were secondary to skin necrosis in 8 out of 14 cases. In this series, we later found that the serious effects of skin necrosis and slough could be prevented by early intervention with a muscle pedicle flap.

Survival

The overall survival time of the patients is 78% in the infected group at 5 years and 70% in the noninfected group. There is no statistically significant difference between the two groups in survival time ($P < 0.98$; log rank test).

Discussion

During the past decade, clinical investigators have reported the efficacy of various chemotherapeutic agents in the treatment of primary and metastatic osteogenic sarcomas

(Freidman and Carter 1972; Jaffe et al. 1978; Pratt et al. 1980; Rosen et al. 1980a, b). Some of these agents included high-dose methotrexate with citrovorum factor rescue, adriamycin, cyclophosphamide, and the combination of bleomycin, cyclophosphamide, dactinomycin and *cis*-platinum. The problem with osteogenic sarcomas in the past has been the impossibility of surgical resection of the primary tumor with adequate free margins without performing an amputation (Rosen et al. 1976). The ability to relieve pain and shrink the primary tumor with chemotherapy in the majority of the patients can decrease the urgency of immediate amputation and afford the surgeon more time to plan definitive treatment.

The multidisciplinary approach to cancer therapy has extended the indications for limb-saving surgery. Patients now receive preoperative chemotherapy before surgical resection in an attempt to improve the results of a standard treatment. In many cases it obviates the need for ablative surgery.

More and more the surgeon is faced with the question of how such treatment will influence morbidity, i.e., wound healing in the postoperative period. In a variety of experimental studies it has been shown that chemotherapy or the combination of chemotherapy and radiation therapy impairs wound healing (Cohen et al. 1975a, b; Mann et al. 1977; Devereux et al. 1979; Desprey and Kiehn 1960; Shastri et al. 1971). However, in no clinical adjuvant trial has significant impairment of wound healing yet been observed.

Adjuvant chemotherapy has been used in many clinical cancer studies, including ovarian, lung, colon, testicular, and gastric tumor protocols. Unfortunately, most clinical reports omit detailed information on wound healing or the timing of administration of drugs in relation to surgery, so that the evaluation of local complications and surgery is difficult (Shields et al. 1977; Higgins et al. 1971; Ansfield et al. 1969; Hattori et al. 1966; Donegan 1974; Fisher et al. 1968). Many of the other chemotherapy protocols are started 2–4 weeks after the surgical procedure, by which time the wound is essentially healed.

In summary, it appears in this series that adjuvant chemotherapy, even given preoperatively, with the last dose given 7 days before surgery, does not seem to have significant adverse effects on wound healing. In only 6% of the patients did amputation have to be performed because of an infection. Wound infection following intensive perioperative chemotherapy does not appear to result in decreased survival time when surgery is performed according to the principles of cancer surgery.

Summary

Reported surgical adjuvant trials in humans have resulted in little clinically significant impairment of wound healing. Such trials are often carried out with subtherapeutic doses or with the drugs administered relatively late in the wound healing process. It is the objective of our study to investigate the effect of intensive pre- and postoperative chemotherapy (BCD, ADR, HD-MTX)[1] on wound healing in patients with osteogenic sarcomas. Wound healing was defined in our study as lack of infection.

In a series of 110 patients with osteogenic sarcomas we analyzed the data of 69 patients with lower extremity lesions: of these, 54 patients had distal femur lesions and 15 had upper tibia and fibula lesions. All the patients underwent en-bloc resections and insertion of a prosthetic device. Pre- and postoperative antibiotics were given routinely.

1 BCD: *B*, bleomycin; *C*, cyclophosphamide; *D*, dactinomycin; *ADR*, adriamycin; *HD-MTX*, high-dose methotrexate

In 80% of our patients (55/69) an uneventful postoperative course was recorded with respect to wound healing. None of these required a secondary operative procedure. Débridement of the wound or débridement of the wound followed by skin grafting had to be performed in 14% (10/69) of the patients. Most of the amputations were performed early in this series of cases. After secondary surgery wound healing was uneventful in most of the patients. No patient died as a consequence of wound infection. Mixed bacterial infections were found in 13/14 patients. No single specific bacterium could be identified. One patient developed a fungal infection (aspergillosis). Eight infections were secondary to skin necrosis. In this series we later found the serious effects of the skin necrosis and slough could be reduced by early intervention with a muscle pedicle flap.

We concluded from our data that (a) intensive pre- and postoperative chemotherapy does not seem to result in a significant impairment of wound healing; (b) in only 6% of the patients was amputation secondary to wound infection or skin necrosis necessary; and (c) wound infection as a consequence of intensive perioperative chemotherapy does not result in a decrease in survival time.

References

Altemeier WA, Barnes BA, Pulaski EJ, Sandusky WR, Burke JF, Clowes GHA (1970) Infections: prophylaxis and management – a symposium. Surgery 67: 369

Ansfield Fl, Korbitz BC, Davis HL, Raminez G (1969) Triple drug therapy in testicular tumors. Cancer 24: 442–446

Cohen SC, Gabelnick HL, Johnson RK, Goldin A (1975a) Effects of antineoplastic agents on wound healing in mice. Surgery 78: 238–244

Cohen SC, Gabelnick HL, Johnson RK, Goldin A (1975b) Effects of cyclophosphamide and adriamycin on the healing of surgical wounds in mice. Cancer 36: 1277–1281

Desprey JD, Kiehn CL (1960) The effects of cytoxan (cyclophosphamide) on wound healing. Plast Reconstr Surg 26: 301–308

Devereux DF, Thibault L, Bonetos J, Brennan MF (1979) The quantitative and qualitative impairment of wound healing by adriamycin. Cancer 43: 932–938

Donegan WL (1974) Extended surgical adjuvant thio-TEPA for mammary carcinoma. Arch Surg 109: 187–192

Fisher B, Ravdin RG, Ausman RK, Slack NH, Moore GE, Noer RS (1968) Surgical adjuvant chemotherapy in cancer of the breast. Ann Surg 168: 337–356

Freidman MA, Carter SK (1972) The therapy of osteogenic sarcoma. Current status and thoughts for the future. J Surg Oncol 4: 482–510

Graves G, Gaaf JH (1980) Effects of chemotherapy on the healing of surgical wounds. Clin Bull MSKCC 10: 4

Guthrie TH, Long PP (1979) Surgical nursing intervention in patients with hematologic malignancies: an overview. Can Nurs: 353

Hattori T, Ito I, Hirata K, Iizuka T, Abe K (1966) Results of combined treatment in patients with cancer of the stomach: palliative gastrectomy, large-dose mitomycin-C, and bone marrow transplantation. Gann 57: 441–451

Higgins GA, Dwight RW, Smith JV, Keehn RJ (1971) Fluorouracil as an adjuvant to surgery in carcinoma of the colon. Arch Surg 102: 339–342

Jaffe N, Frei E, Watts H (1978) High-dose methotrexate in osteogenic sarcoma. A 5-year experience. Cancer Treat Rep 62: 259–264

Mann M, Bednar B, Feit J (1977) Effect of cyclophosphamide on the course of cutaneous wound healing. Neoplasma 24: 487–495

Pratt CB, Howarth C, Ransom JL et al. (1980) High-dose methotrexate alone and in combination therapy for measurable primary or metastatic osteogenic sarcoma. Cancer Treat Rep 64: 11–20

Rosen G, Murphy ML, Huvos AG, Gutierrez M, Marcove RC (1976) Chemotherapy, en bloc resection and prosthetic bone replacement in the treatment of osteogenic sarcoma. Cancer 37: 1–11

Rosen R, Nirenberg A, Juergens H, Caparros B, Huvos AG (1980a) Response of primary osteogenic sarcoma to single agent therapy with high-dose methotrexate with citrovorum factor rescue. In: Nelson JD, Grassi C (eds) Current chemotherapy and infectious disease. Proceedings of the 11th international congress of chemotherapy and the 19th interscience conference on antimicrobial agents and chemotherapy, vol 2. The American Society for Microbiology, Washington, pp 1633–1635

Rosen G, Nirenberg A, Caparros B (1980b) Evaluation of high-dose methotrexate (HDMTX) with citrovorum factor rescue (CFR) single agent chemotherapy in osteogenic sarcoma (OSA). Proc Am Assoc Cancer Res 21: 177

Rosen G, Nirenberg A (1982) Chemotherapy for osteogenic sarcoma: An investigative method – not a recipe. Cancer Treat Rep 66: 1687–1697

Rosen G, Caparros B, Huvos AG, Kosloff C, Nirenberg A, Cacavio A, Marcove RC, Lane J, Mehta B, Urban C (1982) Preoperative chemotherapy for osteogenic sarcoma: selection of postoperative adjuvant chemotherapy based on the response of the primary tumor to preoperative chemotherapy. Cancer 49: 1221–1230

Shamberger RC, Devereux DF, Brennan MF (1981) The effect of chemotherapeutic agents on wound healing. Int Adv Surg Oncol 4: 15–58

Shastri S, Slayton RE, Wolter J, Perlia CP, Taylor SG (1971) Clinical study with bleomycin. Cancer 28: 1141–1146

Shields TW, Humphrey EW, Eastridge CE, Keehn RJ (1977) Adjuvant cancer chemotherapy after resection of carcinoma of the lung. Cancer 40: 2057–2062

Combined-Modality Treatment with Induction Chemotherapy in Locally Advanced Squamous Cell Carcinoma of the Oral Cavity and Oropharynx

R. Abele, W. Lehmann, G. Pipard, and P. Alberto

Hôpital Cantonal Universitaire de Genève, Division d'oncohématologie, Rue Micheli-du-Crest 24, 1211 Genève 4, Switzerland

Introduction

At the University Hospital of Geneva, chemotherapy for recurrent squamous cell carcinoma of the head and neck began in 1972. In a small series of 15 patients, a combination chemotherapy including twice-weekly methotrexate (0.4 mg/kg IV) and bleomycin (30 mg IV) gave 9 objective responses. The median duration of response was only 9 weeks. Toxicity was prominent with this regimen and included 4 early deaths (Broquet et al. 1974). The next trial was initiated with lower weekly doses of methotrexate (0.6 mg/kg IV) and bleomycin (15 mg IV). Partial responses were seen in 13 patients out of 26, with a median duration of 26 weeks. The toxicity of this regimen (Medenica et al. 1976) was considerably lower than that in the initial trial. To optimize the results of chemotherapy in recurrent disease, hydroxyurea at a dose of 1,000 mg/m^2 PO three times per week was added to methotrexate and bleomycin. An overall response rate of 66% including 11 complete remissions, was observed in a total of 32 patients. The mean duration of response was 39 weeks. Toxicity consisted in leukothrombocytopenia in 44% of the patients, gastrointestinal intolerance in 24%, and mucocutaneous toxicity in 19% (Medenica et al. 1981a). In the late 1970s it appeared that cisplatin had a major role in squamous cell carcinoma of the head and neck. After a pilot study of feasibility and tolerance, we took part in a national Swiss cooperative randomized trial (protocol SAKK 10/80) comparing a high dose of cisplatin (100 mg/m^2 on day 2) given with bleomycin (40 mg/m^2 by 48-h continuous infusion) and methotrexate (30 mg/m^2 IV on day 1) administered every 3 weeks against the combination of methotrexate (30 mg/m^2 IV), bleomycin (10 mg/m^2/week IV), hydroxyurea (1,000 mg/m^2 PO 3 times per week) with a medium dose of cisplatin (60 mg/m^2 every 4 weeks). Preliminary analysis of this study showed better results with medium-dose cisplatin than with the high-dose regimen (R. Medenica and J. Wewerka, personal communication).

Induction chemotherapy may yield better results in patients without vascular modifications induced by surgery and/or radiotherapy. Further, patients without prior therapy often have a better performance index and nutrition status than patients with recurrent disease, and could thus have better tolerance to chemotherapy. We investigated the efficacy of the three-drug combination of methotrexate, bleomycin, and hydroxyurea in 67 patients previously untreated for squamous cell carcinoma of the head and neck prior to definite local treatment. With this approach, the overall response rate to chemotherapy was 76%, including 8 complete responses. Toxicity related to treatment was acceptable, with

Recent Results in Cancer Research. Vol. 98

leukothrombocytopenia in 22% of the patients (Medenica et al. 1981b). In spring 1981, we decided to add cisplatin to this three-drug regimen in previously untreated patients to improve local control prior to radiation therapy and/or surgery and postoperative radiation therapy. The feasibility and tolerance to this regimen had already been tested in patients with recurrent disease (R. Medenica and J. Wewerka, personal communication).

Materials and Methods

Patients with histological proof of squamous cell carcinoma of the upper aerodigestive system were included in this trial of induction chemotherapy when curative surgery was judged by a multidisciplinary team of head and neck surgeon, radiation therapist, and medical oncologist to be impossible. All patients had a careful history and physical examination, including panendoscopy and biopsies under general anesthesia. Chest x-rays, complete chemical profile, and hemogram were performed in each patient. Xeroradiography, tomography and/or computed tomography were used when indicated for precise assessment of local tumor extension. All patients were classified according the UICC/TNM system (TNM Classification of malignant tumors 1978).

Chemotherapy consisted of a combination of methotrexate given IV every week at a dose of 22–30 mg/m^2 according to age, performance status, and underlying liver disease; bleomycin 15 mg total dose IV every week; hydroxyurea 1,000 mg/m^2 per day PO every other day. Cisplatin (60 mg/m^2) was given IV once every 4 weeks with short-term pre- and posthydration immediately prior to other drugs on day 1 only. Cisplatin was not given on a randomized basis in this trial. Parenteral chlorpromazine was routinely used as an antiemetic prior to cisplatin administration, and repeated doses were administered when indicated following drug treatment. Patients were seen weekly during induction chemotherapy, clinical examination, hemogram, and renal function tests being performed on each occasion. The length of induction chemotherapy was not uniformly fixed. The response was evaluated after a minimum of 3 weeks of treatment, with the use of standard response criteria (World Health Organization 1979). The duration of chemotherapy was calculated from its initiation to the last day of drug administration. Decisions on definite local treatment were taken cooperatively according to clinical tolerance and response to induction chemotherapy. Survival was calculated from the first day of chemotherapy to death or the cut-off day, using the Kaplan-Meier method (Kaplan and Meier 1958).

Results

Between March 1981 and October 1982, in all 22 consecutive patients were admitted to this trial, 16 male and 6 female. Their median age was 59 years, with a range of 39–75. All male patients had a history of chronic alcohol and tobacco use, but were found to be in an adequate condition for initiation of chemotherapy. No patient had had previous treatment for head and neck cancer.

The primary was found in the oral cavity in 11 patients. Tumors were classified as T4 in four patients, as T3 in four patients, and as T2 in three other patients (UICC stage IV in five patients, stage III in four patients, stage II in two patients). In this group of patients, the primary sites were buccal mucosa (4 patients), lower alveolus (1), tongue (3), and floor of mouth (3). Ten patients had primary tumors in the oropharynx. Lesions were located in the anterior wall in two patients, in the lateral wall in seven patients, and in the superior wall in

one patient. Six patients had T4 tumors, and four had T3 tumors (UICC stage IV 8 patients, stage III 2 patients). The last patient had a T4 paranasal sinus tumor.
The combination of three drugs including methotrexate, bleomycin, and hydroxyurea was given to 8 patients, while 14 patients received quadruple therapy with the same agents plus cisplatin. The median duration of induction chemotherapy was 25 days (range 14–168 days). During this period, a median total dose of 150 mg (range 90–500 mg) methotrexate was given. Median values for bleomycin, hydroxyurea, and cisplatin were 60 mg (range 45–216), 18 g (range 13.5–45), and 143 mg (range 90–510), respectively.
These doses correspond to 88% of the projected dose for methotrexate, 100% for bleomycin, 87% for hydroxyurea, and 100% for cisplatin.
We observed objective responses in five patients: one complete response with complete disappearance of a T4N0 buccal mucosa lesion and four partial responses. The overall response rate to induction chemotherapy was thus only 23% (Table 1). Partial responses were seen in oral cavity primaries (1 patient with a T2N0 and 1 patient with a T3N3 lesion) and in oropharynx primaries (2 patients with T4N1–3 lesions). Responses were observed in primary tumors and in lymph nodes, when affected. Responses were seen in all but one of the patients receiving four-drug combination chemotherapy with cisplatin. Two patients suffered early death, caused by pneumonia and massive tumor hemorrhage. Autopsy in the latter patient revealed only scattered necrobiotic carcinomatous cells in a large oropharyngeal ulcer.
During the chemotherapy period, myelosuppression consisted in leukopenia with a median lowest count of 3.4×10^9/liter (range 2.0–9.6). The median lowest count of thrombocytes was 181×10^9/liter (range 28–376), five patients having values below 100×10^9/liter. Nonhematological toxicity consisted in oral mucositis (3 patients), dermatitis (1 patient), and severe gastrointestinal intolerance (1 patient). It should be noted that this schedule of administration of cisplatin was very well tolerated and that it did not induce prolonged vomiting.
After induction chemotherapy, curative radiation therapy was started in 11 patients on day 49 (median value, range 29–128). Surgery was performed in five patients on day 30 (median value, range 21 to 65) and consisted in radical en-bloc tumor and node removal. All these patients were scheduled for postoperative radiation therapy. This has been achieved in only four patients, since one died from perforation of a duodenal ulcer. In three of these patients, radiation therapy was started within 3 months after initiation of chemotherapy. The fourth patient received radiation therapy with palliative intent 1 year after the operation because of persistence of major swallowing difficulties and late discovery of recurrent disease. External irradiation with tumoricidal doses and one daily fraction was given in nine patients. The multifractionation schedule was administered to six patients. Severe mucositis was observed in five patients during the radiation therapy

Table 1. Response to chemotherapy

Category	No. of patients	%
Complete response	1	5
Partical response	4	18
No change	15	68
Earl death	2	9

period. Six patients did not receive further treatment after induction chemotherapy: three refused further treatment, two died, and one was found to be in too poor a general condition.

With the use of chemotherapy followed by radiation therapy, 4 patients out of 11 were rendered disease free. Chemotherapy, surgery, and radiation therapy yielded the same results in 3 of 4 patients treated in this way. All these patients are alive except one, who had a local relapse and died from his tumor. One patient had only surgery since he died from a non-tumor-related cause. Autopsy of this patient did not reveal persistence of any malignant disease. Of the group of 6 patients who had no further treatment after chemotherapy, only 1 is still alive, without evidence of disease. This patient is a 74-year-old Asiatic woman who had a lesion of the buccal mucosa, probably related to chronic betel nut chewing. Thus only 9 patients of 22 (41%) were rendered disease free in this small series, 7 of whom are still alive with no evidence of disease.

On the other hand, in the 13 patients considered as treatment failures, only 4 patients are still alive, all with evidence of residual disease (Table 2). In this series of patients, the median survival was 46 weeks (Fig. 1).

Discussion

Combination chemotherapy in squamous cell carcinoma of the head and neck has been used at the University Hospital of Geneva since 1972 for recurrent disease. After initial studies with a two-drug combination of methotrexate and bleomycin we reduced drug dosages in the second study, since toxicity was excessive. Better clinical tolerance to chemotherapy and a longer duration of the response were obtained. The addition of a third agent, hydroxyurea, yielded improved results and allowed prolongation of the remissions.

In patients with locally advanced disease of the oral cavity and oropharynx, mainly stage III and IV, we used chemotherapy as the initial treatment to reduce the tumor volume prior to definite local treatment. Combination chemotherapy consisted in three-drug combination of methotrexate, bleomycin, and hydroxyurea or the same agents plus cisplatin. There was no randomization between the two treatments, since there was no intention of comparing the two treatment arms. Cisplatin was added in the latest patients, when it appeared that this agent might have a major impact on the treatment of squamous cell carcinoma of the head and neck.

Table 2. End-results of combined-modality treatment

Type of treatment	No. of patients with NED[a] (alive)	Treatment failures (alive)
Chemotherapy + radiotherapy	4 (3)	7 (3)
Chemotherapy + surgery + postop. radiotherapy	3 (3)	1 (1)
Chemotherapy + surgery	1 (0)	0 (0)
Chemotherapy alone	1 (1)	5 (0)
	9 (7)	13 (4)

[a] No evidence of disease

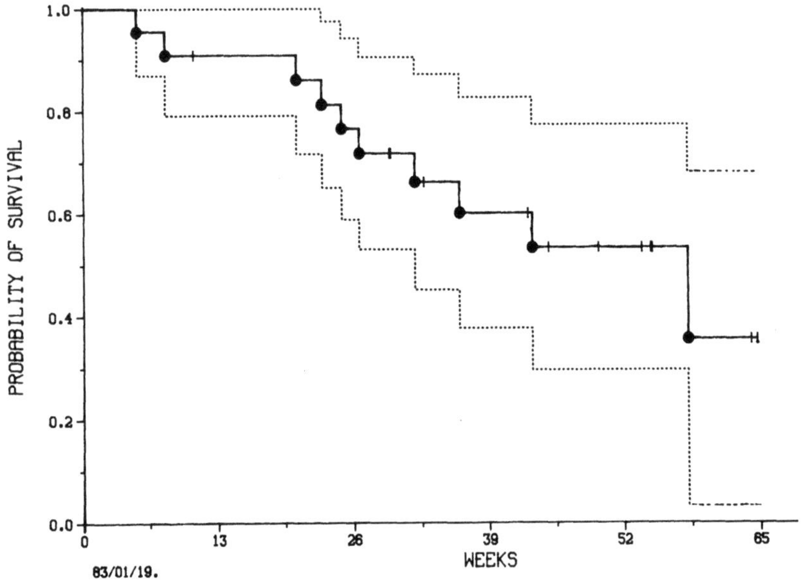

Fig. 1. Survival after combined-modality treatment of epidermoid carcinomas of the head and neck

The present results are disappointing, and indeed the overall response rate to chemotherapy was only 23%, with one complete remission. All the responses except one were seen in patients treated with the cisplatin-containing regimen, indicating that this agent might help to improve results over those possible with regimens not containing cisplatin. For combined-modality treatment the optimum duration of initial chemotherapy is not yet established. Since our patients received chemotherapy only for a short period of time, it is conceivable that a higher response rate might be induced with a longer duration of the chemotherapy period. Nevertheless, results of this short series are inferior to those of our previous study with induction chemotherapy (Medenica et al. 1981b). As patient selection was uniformly conducted, we think that the present results might be related to the site or stage of the disease itself. Further, the small number of patients included in this study does not allow a valid statistical analysis of the response rate.

After induction chemotherapy, 50% of the patients received curative radiation therapy and 18% surgery followed by radiation therapy. No unusual toxicities were noted during these treatment periods, and surgery and/or radiation therapy could be safely conducted in patients with advanced disease who had initially received combination chemotherapy with this regimen.

Patient survival is the end-point of a combined-modality study. Survival of our patients does not differ from that reported recently by other groups in comparable series (Al-Sarraf et al. 1981; Hong et al. 1981; Vogl et al. 1982). There is no evidence of a plateau in the survival curve, indicating the poor probability of definite cure for any subgroup of patients.

In conclusion, locally inoperable squamous cell carcinoma of the oral cavity and oropharynx continues to have a poor prognosis (MacComb et al. 1967; Spiro et al. 1974). Although our present results are inferior to others reported (Al-Sarraf et al. 1981; Hong et al. 1981; Vogl et al. 1982), we intend to continue to use initial chemotherapy in locally advanced head and neck tumors. The value of cisplatin used in combination with methotrexate, bleomycin, and hydroxyurea is now being randomly tested in a Swiss cooperative trial in a larger number of patients. As performance index is one of the major prognostic factors for survival in patients with advanced head and neck cancer (Amer et al. 1979), initial chemotherapy should be administered to patients in good general condition. Improved results might also be seen in patients with less advanced disease than stage III and IV lesions.

Acknowledgements. The authors acknowledge the statistical help and competence of Ms. B. Mermillod, statistician, SAKK Operation Office, CH-1211 Geneva 4, and the secretarial help of Ms. C. Amez-Droz.

References

Al-Sarraf M, Drelichman A, Jacobs J, Kinzie J, Hoschner J, Loh JJK, Weaver A (1981) Adjuvant chemotherapy with cis-platinum, oncovin, and bleomycin followed by surgery and/or radiotherapy in patients with advanced previously untreated head and neck cancer: final report. In: Salmon SE, Jones SE (eds) Adjuvant therapy of cancer III. Grune and Stratton, New York, pp 145–152

Amer MH, Al-Sarraf M, Vaitkevicius VK (1979) Factors that affect response to chemotherapy and survival of patients with advanced head and neck cancer. Cancer 43: 2202–2206

Broquet MA, Jacot-Descombe E, Montandon A, Alberto P (1974) Traitement des carcinomes épidermoïdes oro-pharyngo-laryngés par combinaison de méthotrexate et de bléomycine. Schweiz Med Wochenschr 104: 18–22

Hong WK, Pennacchio J, Shapshay S, Vaughan C, Katz A, Bhutani R, Bromer R, Willett B, Strong S (1981) Adjuvant chemotherapy with cis-platinum and bleomycin infusion prior to definitive treatment for advanced stage III and IV squamous cell head and neck carcinoma. In: Salmon SE, Jones SE (eds) Adjuvant therapy of cancer III. Grune and Stratton, New York, pp 153–160

Kaplan EL, Meier P (1958) Nonparametric estimation from incomplete observations. J Am Statist Assoc 53: 457–481

MacComb WS, Fletcher GH, Healey JE Jr (1967) Intra-oral cavity. In: MacComb WS, Fletcher GH (eds) Cancer of the head and neck. Williams and Wilkins, Baltimore, pp 89–151

Medenica R, Alberto P, Lehmann W (1976) Traitement des carcinomes épidermoïdes oro-pharyngo-laryngés disséminés par combinaison de méthotrexate et de bléomycine à petites doses. Schweiz Med Wochenschr 106: 799–802

Medenica R, Alberto P, Lehmann W (1981a) Combined chemotherapy of head and neck squamous cell carcinomas with methotrexate, bleomycin, and hydroxyurea. Cancer Chemother Pharmacol 5: 145–149

Medenica R, Lehmann W, Pipard G (1981b) Adjuvant chemotherapy of advanced head and neck squamous cell carcinoma, prior to surgery and radiotherapy. Proc AACR/ASCO 22: 430

Spiro RH, Alfonso AE, Farr HW, Strong EW (1974) Cervical node metastasis from epidermoid carcinoma of the oral cavity and oropharynx. Am J Surg 128: 562–567

TNM Classification of malignant tumors (1978) 3rd ed, revised 1982. UICC, Geneva

Vogl SE, Lerner H, Kaplan BH, Coughlin C, McCormick B, Camacho F, Cinberg J (1982) Failure of effective initial chemotherapy to modify the course of stage IV (MO) squamous cancer of the head and neck. Cancer 50: 840–844

World Health Organization (1979) (ed) Handbook for reporting results of cancer treatment, publication no 48, Geneva

Chemotherapy of Squamous Head and Neck Cancer: A Prospective Randomized Trial Comparing cis-Platinum and Bleomycin with Methotrexate and Vindesine

H.-W. von Heyden, M. Schröder, A. Scherpe, J. Borghardt, J.-H. Beyer, G.A. Nagel, H. Gerhartz, B. Foth, E. Kastenbauer, M. Westerhausen, W. Caliebe, H. Rudert, R. Liffers, J. Hofmann, and B. Schneider

Medizinische Einrichtungen der Universität Göttingen, Medizinische Klinik und Poliklinik, Abteilung Hämatologie/Onkologie, Robert-Koch-Strasse 40, 3400 Göttingen, Germany

Introduction

A series of 79 patients with locally inoperable squamous cell carcinoma of the head and neck region were treated from June 1979 to December 1982. The status of inoperability was based on a surgical evaluation indicating that the tumor and/or regional nodes could not be totally resected with curative intent. The aim of this study was to compare an aggressive regimen against a mild one.

Therapy

Figure 1 demonstrates the treatment schedule. Patients were randomized either to regimen A with *cis*-platinum and bleomycin or to regimen B with methotrexate and vindesine. In the case of insufficient response, patients were further treated with the alternative chemotherapy combination (crossover). Whenever possible, surgery and/or radiotherapy was performed in addition to chemotherapy. Patients' characteristics are listed in Table 1, and status with respect to pretreatment, in Table 2. In further prognostic factors such as TNM classification, histological grading, and anatomical regions the two patient groups were nearly homogeneous.

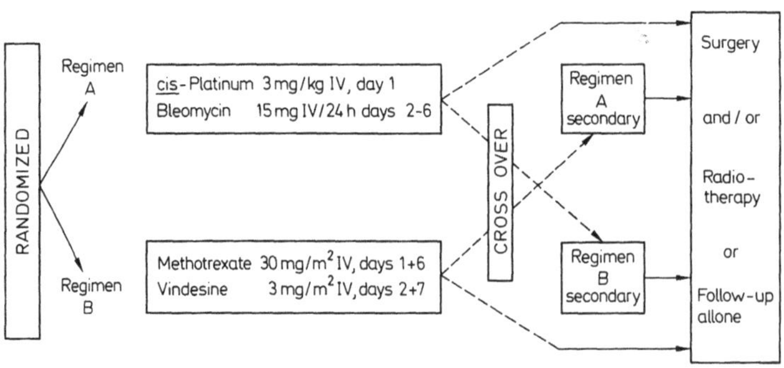

Fig. 1. Treatment schedule

Recent Results in Cancer Research. Vol. 98

Table 1. Patient characteristics

	Regimen A	Regimen B
No of patients	41	38
Median age	53	54
Age range	33–76	34–72
Sex ♂/♀	33/8	29/9

Table 2. Pretreatment status

	Regimen A		Regimen B	
	No of pts.	%	No of pts.	%
Not pretreated	27	66	24	63
Pretreated[a]	14	34	14	37
Op + RT	12		13	
Op	1		–	
RT	1		–	
RT + CH	–		1	

[a] *Op*, surgery; *RT*, radiotherapy; *CH*, chemotherapy

Table 3. Response to chemotherapy

	Regimen A		Regimen B		Crossover to A		Crossover to B	
	No.	%	No.	%	No.	%	No.	%
CR	0		1	3	1	6	0	
PR	24	59	10	26	5	29	0	
MR	10	24	11	29	5	29	0	
NC	6	15	10	26	3	18	2	20
PD	1	2	6	16	3	18	8	80
	41		38		17		19	

Results

The response to chemotherapy shows (Table 3) that regimen A was superior to regimen B. The major response rate in A was 59%, as against 29% in B. These results were further supported by those in the crossover group. *cis*-Platinum and bleomycin induced complete and partial remissions in 6 of 17 patients who were resistant to methotrexate and vindesine. In addition, no response was observed in the patients resistant to *cis*-platinum and bleomycin when further treated with methotrexate and vindesine. Therefore, crossover from regimen A to regimen B was discontinued.

Regarding the major response rate, the pretreatment status may be of more prognostic importance for the less aggressive combination with methotrexate and vindesine than for

Table 4. Response to chemotherapy according to preatment status

	Previous treatment				No prior treatment			
	Regimen A		Regimen B		Regimen A		Regimen B	
	No.	%	No.	%	No.	%	No.	%
CR	0		0		0		1	4
PR	7	50	2	14	17	63	8	33
MR	2	14	3	22	8	30	8	33
NC	4	29	7	50	2	7	3	13
PD	1	7	2	14	0		4	17
	14		14		27		24	

Table 5. Response to chemotherapy according to anatomical regions

	Oral cavity		Oropharynx		Larynx		Hypopharynx	
	No.	%	No.	%	No.	%	No.	%
CR	0		1	4	0		0	
PR	7	54	9	40	5	38	9	36
MR	4	31	6	26	6	46	5	20
NC	2	15	6	26	1	8	7	28
PD	0		1	4	1	8	4	16
	13		23		13		25	

the more aggressive one (Table 4). Partial remissions were achieved with regimen A in 50% of patients pretreated with surgery and/or radiotherapy, as against 15% with regimen B. The partial remission rates in patients not pretreated were 63% with A and 37% with B. Better chemotherapy results can therefore be expected in those patients not pretreated by surgery and/or radiotherapy. This even seems to be true for the categories of minor response, no change, and progressive disease.

Regarding other prognostic factors, patients with low histological differentiation did not show any difference in response to those with poorly or well-differentiated tumors. Tumor size and nodal status also exhibited no influence on response to chemotherapy. However, with reference to anatomical regions it seems that patients with tumor of the oral cavity or oropharynx respond better than those with tumors of the larynx or hypopharynx (Table 5).

Side-effects of chemotherapy are listed in Table 6. *cis*-Platinum and bleomycin were generally less well tolerated than methotrexate and vindesine. The latter combination was given without admitting the patients to hospital.

Table 7 shows the results of surgery and/or radiotherapy following primary chemotherapy (no pretreatment with either of these procedures). The results of surgery and/or radiotherapy are referred to those obtained with the preceding chemotherapy. The

Table 6. Side-effects

	cis-Platinum/ bleomycin	Methotraxate/ vindesine
Nausea/vomiting	93%	17%
Hair-loss	60%	44%
Stomatitis	2%	6%
Polyneuropathy	10%	6%
Ototoxicity	7%	–
Nephropathy	35%	4%
Lung fibrosis	19%	–
Leukopenia	22%	31%
Thrombopenia	12%	21%
Anemia	17%	19%
Liver toxicity	2%	15%
Others	21%	17%

Table 7. Response to further treatment by surgery (*OP*) and or radiotherapy (*RT*) in comparison with response to previous chemotherapy (*CH*) in patients with no pretreatment before chemotherapy

$n = 5$	CH		OP		$n = 16$	CH		RT		$n = 23$	CH		OP+RT	
	No.	%	No.	%		No.	%	No.	%		No.	%	No.	%
CR	1	20	4	80	CR	1	6	4	25	CR	0		18	79
PR	2	40	0		PR	5	31	4	25	PR	17	74	3	13
MR	2	40	0		MR	7	44	0		MR	6	26	1	4
NC	0		1	20	NC	2	13	0		NC	0		0	
PD	0		0		PD	1	6	8	50	PD	0		1	4

therapeutic procedure for operation or radiotherapy or both was decided individually. Therefore, it must be stressed that patients were not randomized. Several patients were unwilling or unable to undergo surgical procedures. However, whenever performance status allowed or whenever technically possible, operation was performed. After careful consideration of these results it is our personal opinion that radiotherapy alone should not be performed.

For patients with head and neck cancer survival curves are more important than response rates. Our survival analysis is not yet finished, but there is no difference in median survival between regimen A and regimen B. The median survival is about 11 months for the nonpretreated patients and 7 months for those previously treated. There is a significant difference in the crossover group. Patients resistant to A and treated further with regimen B had a median survival of less than 3 months. However, patients resistant to B and treated further with A have a median survival of 9 months ($P = 0.02$).

Conclusions

In terms of remission rates *cis*-platinum (DDP) and bleomycin (BLM) is more effective than methotrexate (MTX) and vindesine (VDS).
Patients with inadequate response to MTX and VDS can in addition be successfully treated with DDP and BLM. However, patients with inadequate response to DDP and BLM cannot expect any further benefit from MTX and VDS. Therefore, crossover from DDP and BLM to MTX and VDS should not be continued.
Pretreatment status (surgery and/or radiotherapy) may be of less prognostic value for the more aggressive combination of DDP and BLM than for the less aggressive one of MTX and VDS. In patients who had not been pretreated the results of chemotherapy were better.
With regard to histological grading, tumor size, and nodal status there is no evident difference in response rates between the chemotherapy modalities. Tumors of the oral cavity or oropharynx respond more favorably to chemotherapy than those of the larynx and hypopharynx.
Preliminary survival analysis reveals no difference between regimen A and regimen B in respect of the prognostic factors. Analysis of subsets shows that patients treated by crossover from regimen B to regimen A live significantly longer than those treated by crossover from regimen A to regimen B.
Chemotherapy is indicated in patients with locally inoperable tumors. In the case of tumor reduction, additional radical surgery and eventually radiotherapy must be performed to give a chance of cure, since this does not seem to be possible with chemotherapy alone.

Summary

Present Status and Future Prospects in Perioperative Chemotherapy

U. Metzger, F. Largiadèr, and H.-J. Senn

Chirurgische Onkologie, Departement Chirurgie, Universitätsklinik, 8091 Zürich, Switzerland

For methodological reasons a clear distinction should be made between *preoperative* and *perioperative* chemotherapy. Preoperative and perioperative chemotherapy have somewhat different goals. *Preoperative* chemotherapy may have the advantage of providing markers for responsiveness. This might be considered as one of the end-points, as it has been by Rosen in osteogenic sarcoma. In selected cases, resectability might be enhanced by preoperative chemotherapy. With this therapeutic approach, we lose the ability to stage adequately at the time of tumor diagnosis. If we can ultimately show a clear advantage in terms of overall survival it is not really necessary to know in fine detail what we are doing. The problem is that the risks always become apparent first (early toxicity, lack of response, inability of adequate staging), before we have any idea of how much weight we can put on the benefit side of the scale. In deciding between preoperative and perioperative chemotherapy another problem is the additional length of time for which a patient is eligible before the exclusion criteria apply; an example is given with reference to the modalities of radiation and surgery: preoperative radiation therapy for rectal cancer may have some benefit for local control, but this benefit is useless if small liver or peritoneal metastases are detected at laparotomy.

In a multimodality treatment program, the patient's – and sometimes even the doctor's – compliance for the second modality varies, depending on the modality given first. For this reason, the most effective treatment should be given first. On the other hand, preoperative chemotherapy may have the advantage of tumor shrinkage and enhanced resectability. In addition, if surgery is adequately timed in the recovery phase of chemotherapy, even an immunostimulatory rebound effect has been claimed for preoperative chemotherapy. However, there are no convincing data so far to prove that preoperative chemotherapy significantly increases overall survival in randomized comparison to surgery alone. Many promising results obtained in phase II trials now need confirmation by randomized phase III studies.

Before entering on *perioperative,* i.e., early postoperative, adjuvant chemotherapy trials, a rational way to proceed should be decided upon. First of all, the chemotherapy under consideration should be effective in at least 40% of cases in the advanced disease situation. Then, this chemotherapy could be tested for so-called conventionally timed adjuvant chemotherapy. If an advantage is found for this type of adjuvant treatment the results might be optimized by moving the adjuvant therapy closer to the operation and evaluating it as perioperative chemotherapy, as in the current Ludwig Breast Cancer Study. This methodological approach can be considered as a general rule, but there are some

Recent Results in Cancer Research. Vol. 98

objections: Nissen-Meyer and his group have clearly shown that a single-drug treatment can be active, provided this adjuvant therapy is given as soon as possible after surgery, even if this treatment is quite ineffective in advanced disease. Experimental data strongly support the hypothesis that a drug or a drug combination is more effective with a smaller body burden of tumor stem cells. In a single animal, the same treatment can lead to curative reduction of small body burdens of small numbers of cells – micrometastatic foci – while yielding no measurable reduction in the body burden of a large mass, probably due to higher exposure of tumor cells to lethal drug concentrations in microscopic disease than in a large tumor mass, where the vasculature is poor. In the near future, in vitro chemosensitivity testing could become a valuable approach to reveal drugs that might be active against microscopic deposits while possibly ineffective in advanced disease. On the other hand, if there is a highly active drug combination for advanced disease (e.g., testicular cancer) no adjuvant treatment is needed.

The second point to be considered is the treatment of recurrent disease if patients have already received the most effective treatment in the adjuvant situation. How do these patients respond to the same chemotherapy in relapse? Sparse data are available on this topic, and probably adjuvant chemotherapy impairs a secondary response to the same treatment. But the object of adjuvant chemotherapy is to increase the cure rate, and if this is indeed achieved there is a lesser need for chemotherapy of recurrent disease.

The third and most important aspect of moving adjuvant chemotherapy closer to the operation is the increased toxicity. There is experimental evidence that many drugs influence wound healing and wound breaking strength. But it was unanimously stated by the surgeons present that wound healing is not the basic problem of toxicity. More importance attaches to the postoperative complications in drug-induced pancytopenia. Surgical complications in lung, stomach, or large-bowel cancer surgery are not as rare as they are in breast cancer, and they are certainly more difficult to handle if they occur during drug-induced immunosuppression. Drugs could be selected for not having bone marrow toxicity or those chosen that do not influence wound healing. In addition, the start of perioperative chemotherapy could be determined individually, because some patients will recover quickly from surgery while others need much more time, so that the criteria for starting perioperative chemotherapy could vary according to clearance of atelectasis, clearance of ileus, removal of drainage, etc. However, from the methodological viewpoint such a trial will be anything but clear-cut, and very difficult to evaluate. Nevertheless, if, for example in the Ludwig V trial, the end-results are the same, so that a 1-month course of perioperative chemotherapy has as good an effect as 6 months of conventionally timed adjuvant chemotherapy, the patient can be spared 5 months' exposure to toxic effects. One of the difficult issues of perioperative chemotherapy is that the surgeons are now becoming familiar with a kind of toxicity that the medical oncologist is used to dealing with. For the benefit of the patient it may be reasonable: the same therapeutic result or even better with 5 months' less cytotoxic therapy. Probably the surgeons should be ready to compromise by accepting a slightly higher level of postoperative morbidity.

This acceptance could certainly be increased if markers were available to measure residual tumor burden. In the adjuvant situation this would allow a distinction between the patients who are really cured from the very beginning and those who are not cured by surgery alone. While ever such markers are not available the physician should first avoid unneccessary toxicity and harm to the patient who is potentially cured by surgery alone.

The Symposium highlighted the attractiveness of combining local and systemic treatment. It clearly showed the urgent need for randomized, controlled clinical studies to determine the ultimate role of both preoperative and perioperative chemotherapy. We have just entered a new field of combined-modality therapy with chemotherapy given around the time of surgery, and a lot of clinical research work remains to be done, the most positive impact being the closer cooperation of medical and surgical oncologists.

Subject Index

MIX
Papier aus verantwortungsvollen Quellen
Paper from responsible sources
FSC® C105338

If you have any concerns about our products,
you can contact us on
ProductSafety@springernature.com

In case Publisher is established outside the EU,
the EU authorized representative is:
Springer Nature Customer Service Center GmbH
Europaplatz 3, 69115 Heidelberg, Germany

Printed by Libri Plureos GmbH
in Hamburg, Germany